extreme clinic

An Outpatient Doctor's Guide to the
Perfect 7-Minute Visit

D1596323

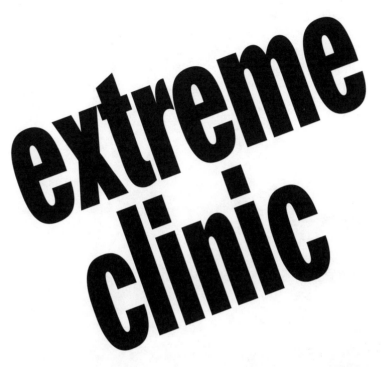

An Outpatient Doctor's Guide to the Perfect 7-Minute Visit

Tom Laurence, MD

Staff Neurologist
VA Illiana Health Care System
Danville, Illinois
Assistant Professor of Internal Medicine
Internal Medicine Residency Program
University of Illinois College of Medicine
Urbana, Illinois

HANLEY & BELFUS
An Affiliate of Elsevier

HANLEY & BELFUS, INC.
An Affiliate of Elsevier

The Curtis Center
Independence Square West
Philadelphia, Pennsylvania 19106

Library of Congress Control Number: 2003107919

**Extreme Clinic: An Outpatient Doctor's Guide
to the Perfect 7-Minute Visit**　　　　　ISBN 1-56053-603-9

Printed in the United States of America

Last digit is the print number:　9　8　7　6　5　4　3　2　1

For Pat,
with whom it happens

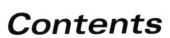

Contents

Introduction

Around midnight of the third year into our craft and sullen art comes a terrifying epiphany, when we know for absolute certain that we've been duped. The patient sitting gowned before us turns and utters sweetly the shattering words: "Doctor, everything I eat turns to gas, my teeth itch, and it feels like an octopus is sucking my brains out...." We realize in those ten seconds that all our time devoted to the formal mysticism of membrane potentials, the crypts of Lieberkuhn, and the fields of Forel would have been better spent snorkeling in Bora Bora or reading Baudelaire in a sidewalk cafe in Montmartre.

Medical school doesn't teach us how to practice medicine. Maybe five decades ago, when our skilled trade was more apprenticeship, we *did* pick up a few tips from the old docs we followed around. No HMOs, no malpractice, no third parties, and no paperwork gave us a lot of free time to learn how to wrangle patients. Low tech, no pharmaceutical giants, and no Internet helped, too. And back then we had all that paternalism and meritocratic mystique on our side. We could spend hours with a patient and no one bothered us or dared ask what we were doing. We reigned and basked in such a protected glory.

It's over. We're labor now. We follow algorithms, order techno tests, do a lot of procedures, and fill out inane forms—crossing our fingers and hoping we do get paid and don't get sued.

The patient has receded, and as we've lost our mystique, so have we lost freedom and charisma. Front-line primary care medicine has drifted toward burger flipping. Our physician autonomy, the room to study our patients and work with them up close, has dwindled. What can we do to take back our territory, that special and exciting domain of practicing medicine?

I started looking for solutions in the late 80s when it was already clear that doctoring had become managed and physicians were no longer calling the shots. Time spent with the patient had already plummeted, the work-up and therapy had become cookbook, and all concerned were watching the clock and the bottom line. Disenchantment was setting in, and physicians were having a hard time putting their fingers on how it had all gone wrong.

In 1990 I spent a year of Fridays in the depths of the Firestone Library at Princeton University reading metamedicine. What is disease, what is suffering, what do doctors actually *do*? My study overlapped cultural anthropology, the history and philosophy of medicine, sociology, and economics. The following year, returning to the clear light of day, I started dissecting what goes into an outpatient visit. What's the agenda for a specific visit? How do doctors and patients act together? How do they move in and out of the examining room? What goes on in their dialog? What about personal space? What *really* gets done in the clinic?

Next, I completely overhauled how I ran a busy outpatient service. Within months the 20-minute exam had become 7 minutes. The patients were more satisfied, more was getting accomplished, and I still felt fresh when the last patient of the day was headed for home.

My colleagues were intrigued, and I began to give informal workshops on what I called the guerilla clinic, unconventional medical practice. The ponderous complete histories and physicals were scrapped, and the S.O.A.P. approach was completely gutted. Open-ended questions were phased out, and benevolent interruption of the patient's narrative was phased in.

I had also been watching people in motion out in the world, looking at ergonomics, analyzing how the folks at

Jiffy Lube and Pizza Hut did their thing. I drew from film directing, theater, time-motion studies, and Samurai strategy. I borrowed tricks from the mentors and colleagues who had done a few things right, from surgeons at their best, and from the dialog techniques of psychoanalysts. And I looked most closely at what family practitioners and general internists were consistently doing wrong.

When I joined the faculty of the University of Illinois College of Medicine in 1991, I started teaching my collection of streamlined skills to medical students as tutorials, later adding the techniques to my rotation for residents in the university's internal medicine program. I put the basics into a lecture format, added a Q & A session, and *Extreme Clinic* was born. The rest has been ten years of fine-tuning, continual revision, and pure joy.

Extreme Clinic is for every doctor who sees more than one patient a day. It is for medical students who want to take all that burden off their shoulders and for residents and fellows who are going to be out in the real world real soon, practicing their own style of medicine without those nitpicking attendings. And it is also for the attendings, who might want to take a look at how they practice, mend their ways, and have delightful, longer lives for themselves.

Extreme Clinic gives us a way to save time, spirit, and ATP. It opens up a path back to the sheer pleasure of being a physician. And it has given me the time and energy to write the book so that I can share my secrets with you.

Tom Laurence, MD
Urbana, Illinois

Your Mission

Put down the *New England Journal* that just arrived. It's time to glance at your appointment book, take a peek at who's in the waiting room, and start seeing patients. There's a little old lady with two shopping bags and a walker, clutching a crumpled list of thirty new symptoms. There's a hypertensive diabetic with pitting edema. The gloomy man in the corner looks awfully depressed. Your asthmatic is wheezing and so is the dusky smoker with the barrel chest. At least one of your flock is harboring a carcinoma that won't show up for a decade. Another doesn't know it, but she has a tight coronary artery stenosis and feels just great. When the day is over, each of these people and a dozen or so more will have been doctored and sent their separate ways. Your mission, should you choose to accept it, is to make each visit quick, effective, and dedicated. No patient will feel rushed or treated as a number, and you will leave your office without a sense of exhaustion. You are about to embark on a course of nonconventional patient care, the world of the Extreme Clinic.

Sooner or later you will be abandoning the traditional approach to the patient. It might as well be now. You will trim, edit, and gently guide the delivery of the presenting complaint, at the same time laying on hands. You will combine history taking with physical examination, beginning your palpation of body parts within the first minutes of the visit. The disposition and an agenda for the next visit are both in the works from the beginning. You will not be waiting passively for a diagnosis to evolve from some invisible prophetic machine. Take comfort and strength in knowing that ultimately the practice of medicine is a study of the patient. The rest is style.

As in elective surgery, the secret of an effective clinic visit is a detailed plan. Unknown to the next patient, you have taken a 30-second break to be alone with his chart before closing it and entering the room. In that moment you have reviewed what happened last time—looking over test results, medications, and a reminder to ask about his prize orchids and the trip he was planning to Majorca. That peaceful moment, spent alone with your patient's record, sharpens the image of his illness and his persona—concentrating all your years of training on one human being. It is a moment of great power, a meditation before walking onto the stage, the mental focus before the starting gun:

"Good morning Mr. Corpus. Has that Isordil made any difference in how often you get an angina attack? The last time I saw you the blood pressure was 170/100. Roll up your sleeve and let's see what it is today. How was Majorca? How do you like the new humidifier you installed in your greenhouse?"

Keep moving and allow no empty airtime.

A colleague down the hall had a habit of opening every visit with "Have I ever seen you before?" Aside from instantly creating an aura of not knowing and not caring, he was wasting time. Every encounter became a starting-all-over. Without a clear and detailed idea of why your patient is here and what dispositions his illness may generate, you are doomed to the impotence of "How have you been feeling?" and its dreaded consequences, "Not very well, Doctor—and I've made a list here of all my problems."

Have a nice day.

Picture you and your patient walking through today's visit to a logical outcome—a clean break. On what notes will we begin and end? Your patient thinks you've been working on his case since your last encounter. And so you have.

Doctors are more effective and more comfortable dealing with diseases than with their patients' stories. Pathologists and surgeons smile knowingly to themselves as they listen to the tales of their brothers and sisters in family practice and psychiatry: "Then she started telling me it felt like a jet liner roaring through her head." A cystic astrocytoma on the CT scan of your patient's brain carries a comfortable familiarity that vanishes when you enter the private domain of its messenger: "I started hearing a little tune and smelled violets, and then the carpet started looking so thick, and I'd wake up on the floor with blood on my cheek."

Aim to separate the patient's morbid anatomy from her suffering every time you see her. Set up algorithms to track the natural history of your patients' diseases—behind the scenes—while devoting that intensive looking, listening, and feeling to the unique mystery of the person in front of you. Let your staff know that they will be following a certain cluster of trends in every diabetic patient, in everyone with atherosclerosis, in all patients who have had seizures. A loyal technician with the right software can babysit disease while you're concentrating on the illness.

Inside your head are an actuary and a public health physician, looking at your practice from afar, putting your patients' destinies into the context of probability and chance. The personality of the illness takes shape through your dialog, while the personality of disease develops through your lifelong studies. Although you may never know the inner nature of your patient's illness, how she senses her body and its idiosyncrasies, you can analyze her organs' changes and their various fates—and you can do it in private, as you have through all those years of long nights reading. There may be nothing you can do about that jet liner, but the two packs of cigarettes a day, the lipids, and the blood pressure can keep you both busy until death doth you part.

Some days your agenda fails and the visit falters. The disease has thrown you a curve, or the patient brings you a bundle of suffering you hadn't predicted. A metastasis just showed up in a man who thought himself cured. Your stable MS patient found out yesterday her husband is divorcing her; she's here today with double vision. The charming woman you put on amiodarone last month looked in the mirror this morning and noticed she's turning blue. She is fuming and pacing back and forth in your waiting room talking to her attorney on a cell phone.

Don't panic! Take a deep breath, turn on that Platonic circuitry you're getting paid for, meditate (as always) for a moment or two with the chart, and remind yourself that there's no other profession that gets itself into such a pack of trouble. There is no etching in stone telling you to heal, fix, and cure all day long. Sit back—listen to the music of the patient's words as though you're playing a duet. Observe her gestures with the eyes of a hawk, placing you and your needs beyond the horizon. Capture the essence of doctoring.

You and I, dear doctor, are going out in that waiting room to bring our patients in one by one. We're going to give them our best, making sense, when we can, of their bodies and their pathos. Together we'll do the whole clinic for the day, for we have nothing else planned and nowhere else to be.

What They Want

Some years ago a patient confided, "I care about two things in a doctor. He looks me in the eye when I'm talking to him, and his hands are warm when he touches my body. If he also happens to know some medicine, that's a plus." This is the best-case scenario, the patient made in heaven. What makes clinical practice tricky is that the patient's agenda, needs, illness and disease are in constant flux. Your colleague tells you that she extracted a history of A, found B and C on exam, ordered D and E, and summed it up for her patient in F. But he was simply furious, stormed out of her office, and never went back. It was the wrong stuff, the wrong patient, the wrong time, and just maybe the wrong doctor.

Ask yourself before, during, and after each visit, *"Why is he here? Why is he really here? What are we doing? Where are we headed? What can we achieve with a return appointment?"* It's easy to go with the flow and have him come back in three months for a "routine" visit, for no particular reason, but what then? Will he likely have had enough symptoms for the two of you to talk about? Will his disease have advanced enough by then to make it worth a new look?

The patient wants to have "been-to-the-doctor" according to her own standards for that ritual. She wants to get in to see you quickly and to get out quickly. No matter how charismatic and omniscient you may be, she has better things to do today than hanging around your clinic, or you can hope. Be on time and reflect not a flicker of haste.

Your patient wants a moment of clarity and affirmation in the midst of the chaos of daily life. She expects privacy in direct proportion to intimacy. Create an oasis for her through meticulous attention to isolating her from the sight, sound, and presence of others. A warm, quiet, spotless, well-lit room is essential.

Your patient wants to be taken seriously, and to be able to plead her case without prejudice, labeling, or rush to judgment. She is paying for your unbiased gaze.

"I know what you're going to say, Doctor—that I need to start exercising and lose a few pounds."

"I wasn't, but I'm curious as to why you thought so." You may have been tempted, but your recommendations can wait awhile. Timing is critical.

We all want to be thought unique. Your patient wants you to see something in him separate from the world of commercials for pain pills.

"I know you see a lot of people with headaches, Doc, and I know you listen to a lot of stories." No, never before, nothing like this, certainly not yours.

We hear that patients want "their own" doctors. What then is this creature called *my own doctor*? The mundane aspects of health care—handing out cards to rub with feces, checking blood sugars and pressures, and ordering panels of tests—can be taken care of by an enthusiastic high school dropout at the front desk. These are *I've been to the clinic* maneuvers. What, then, do *you* do that is so special?

You remember her as though you had grown up together, "Mrs. Darling, when I saw you back in March for that urinary tract infection, you mentioned that your sister Ellen had some kidney problems about ten years ago, glomerulonephritis as I recall?" Committing dates, places, names, and numbers to short-term recall adds to your charisma. *How in the world did she remember all that?* Because I'm your doctor and it's my job to know all about you, that's how.

"Remember when you first came to see me three years ago with blurred vision feeling so exhausted and Ann checked your blood sugar? It was 600 as I recall. You were pretty sick, and you had some strong feelings about starting insulin because of your mother's experience."

You're sensitive, Doc, and you know the difference between diabetes mellitus and personal memories.

"You don't like taking Tegretol, do you?" We've talked about your sense of giving up control, and how you skip doses when you haven't had an aura for awhile. I know what you've been through with your seizures. I remember your using the phrase "love-hate relationship" to describe how you feel about your auras."

Your exact quote reflects not only that you really *were* listening, but that you respect her experience. You know her style, her idiosyncrasies, and her individuality.

Think Disposition

As psychoanalysts know better than any of us, the ultimate goal of the doctor-patient relationship is termination. Surgeons are good at this too. How often do you hear anyone talking about doctoring with his surgeon unless he's going back to get the stitches out? We, the non-analysts and non-surgeons, can use end-oriented strategy just as well. Think outcome. As today's visit begins you are already at work on winding things up. On what note and with what words will you be parting? How will you dispose of the body?

Conventional teaching dictates that the course of our encounter will emerge from the patient's opening words, the presenting complaint. From a few phrases of history, a physical examination, and some labs, we are supposed to script a coherent minidrama. That may be true in the perfect world of textbook medicine, but what can *really* be done in the seven to ten minutes of today's fast-paced clinic?

If you're lucky the patient tells you as soon as she enters the examining room that in the past few days she has become yellow, has been passing urine the color of dark tea, and feels a pain in her right upper quadrant. Such is the theoretical presentation of disease in a Platonic clinic. But what if the opening lines get snagged on "Everything I eat turns to gas," or feelings of organs sinking through the floor of the pelvis, or something wobbling around in the brain? Our beloved quasi-scientific biomedicine, which works so well in the comfort of textbook and armchair, just isn't built to handle such primeval laments. And the clock is ticking.

As an extreme doctor it is your job, not the patient's, to choose the theme of the day and the agenda for the visit. Abandon "How have you been?," which yields the dreaded

"Not so well. I've made a list here of the symptoms I've been having since my last appointment."

Instead, begin the dialog with system-specific and disorder-specific questioning: "How many nitroglycerin tablets have you been using per week since you started Isordil?"

As you move closer to your patient, combine opening questions with physical examination of pertinent organs. Laying on the hands accompanies rather than follows your dialog. Begin touching and using your instruments within the first 60 seconds of opening the session. You can be squeezing the ankles, feeling a pulse, and putting your stethoscope on the chest, all the while asking about shortness of breath, chest pain, and response to medication. For whatever reason or quirk of intuition, you've chosen today's episode to be the fine-tuning of cardiopulmonary stuff. The elapsed time is about five minutes, and you're heading into the home stretch:

"We're going to be stopping in two or three minutes. Why don't we increase the Lasix and recheck your electrolytes and digoxin level. I'd like you to keep monitoring your blood pressure and weight at home and call me Tuesday to let me know how you're doing. I won't need to see you back in the office until the end of April. I've done most of the talking today, do you have any questions?"

You and your patient have collaborated in updating the clinical picture, and plans for the next appointment are already afoot. Leaving a patient's questions to the end grants them greater importance. Since her questions and concerns will be following a visceral and detail-oriented scrutiny of her present condition, they stand a better chance of being more introspective and more concise. Be specific in your replies as you prepare for departure, one hand on her shoulder and the other on the doorknob, physically removing her body and baggage:

"I'll be talking with you on Tuesday, Ms. Pathos, and we'll be seeing each other in April."

People and Patients

It is a dangerous peculiarity of doctoring that we grant patienthood by default to just about anybody who turns up on our doorstep. *If you've got a complaint that sounds medical, then you're a patient, my patient.* Wrong.

All patients are people but all people aren't patients. We've spent more than a couple of minutes asking a drug rep about his presenting complaint, granting him full patienthood, before realizing he had simply made it through the filters of the front desk to pitch his new pill. A young woman complaining of "bladder problems" wound up getting asked about double vision and ataxia before we realized she mistook *neuro* for *uro* and simply needed Septra for a UTI. Another five minutes and she would have got a needle in her back and an MRI of her head and spinal cord.

The man at the table next to you in the restaurant starts slurring his words and drops his fork. You can't help noticing that his mouth is drooping. He's having a TIA. *That's a patient having a TIA.* Having a TIA, yes—your patient, no. You may well become a good Samaritan and go over to his table and do your doctor thing, but you're entering his world as though you're an anthropologist. He hasn't "come to you."

All diseases live in people who don't become patients until they come to see us, entering into the weird and often unspoken contract of the doctor-patient duo. Sometimes the transformation slips right past us. *A moment ago I looked out my office window and noticed a man with a limp in the parking lot. Now he's in my waiting room, now in the examining room. All of a sudden this stranger is my patient.* The clinic automatically bestows patienthood. Pay attention to this invisible metamorphosis.

We spend two years studying disease detached from patient. Then we're plunged into the world of people-with-complaints, a rude awakening. So eager are we to have patients of our own that we begin to skip the person-as-case-study and go directly to "She's my patient, she's mine." Be careful what you wish for, dear doctor.

Go out into the street. Go out among the masses. See people. Stare at them and study them. Watch and listen and record their habits and locomotions in your brain, building up your database of normal and not so normal. Sooner or later you'll start spotting the Parkinson people, the ones in chemotherapy, the goiter lady in the mall. There's a man with a wheelchair who doesn't need a wheelchair. Over there a cirrhotic's belly hanging out over the belt. These are people, not patients. They are, at the moment, the human race, and you are merely a keen observer, a doctor perhaps, but certainly not their doctor. What a relief!

When we first start seeing human beings with complaints on our own turf, namely in the clinic we have to pay rent for, we are simply overjoyed. Use a little restraint. If a candidate for patienthood seems like more than you want to handle, spend a preliminary visit looking at the two of you—goals, expectations, and styles. Once you're stuck with each other, running off to Reno for a quickie divorce isn't an option.

The Agenda

The agenda is what you're going to do with the next patient. It is the heart and soul of the Extreme Clinic. It is your opening move and the game plan to follow. It is your script, your stage directions, your lights, camera, and action all in one. You will always create an agenda *before* you set foot in the examining room.

You'll put together the agenda from a bit or piece of your total knowledge of the patient, the trend of her disease, and whatever new complaint she may have presented to your staff at the front desk. Let's say, for example, that your agenda is *delivering the diagnosis of carcinoma of the uterus and referral to a surgeon:*

"Good morning, Ms. Fallop. I'd like to show you the CT films of your pelvis. Your blood tests and chest x-ray were normal. Let me get the films up on the view box. Come over here where you can see better."

If the agenda is *decreasing frequency of asthma attacks,* then you might enter the room, stethoscope in hand, where the patient has already been gowned, place your arm over your patient's scapula, and open with:

"Good morning, Ms Alveole. Let me listen to that chest. How many puffs of albuterol have you been using this past week?"

If the agenda is *management of acute on recurrent renal colic* then:

"Good morning Mr. Nefrose. You passed some kidney stones two years ago November, didn't you. Show me with one finger where that pain is and where it goes. Is this tender? Have you had any blood in your urine? Any chills or fever? Do you think this is different from two years ago?"

The agenda is a path to a disposition. It contains a tentative diagnosis and a tentative course of action. The agenda is your educated hunch based on the story and data to date, and based on the way diseases play themselves out over time. The agenda never starts from scratch and it *never* begins with casting out a net for a presenting complaint. The agenda will *never* begin with:

"Good morning, Ms. Spode. Why are you here today? How may I help you? What's going on with you? How have you been feeling? I understand you've been having some problems with your breathing? Would you like to tell me more about it?"

You don't have the time or energy to recreate the entire history of western medicine with your patients, forever starting all over as though for the first time. Nor do you want to dilute the richness of detail in an acute problem by drifting off into the land of general review of systems. Begin with the specific and stay with the specific. Expand to the general only when absolutely necessary. And when you do, go for detail there too.

Your nurse has told you that Mr. Iktal, whom you've seen twice before, has come in today after phoning to let her know that he had a seizure last night. He's never mentioned seizures in the past. You enter the room, place your hands on his head, and ask him to stick out his tongue for a second, and get ready with your ophthalmoscope:

"Good Morning, Mr. Iktal. Going back over your whole lifetime, have you ever had *any* kind of blackout, or spell, or seizure, or fit, or loss of consciousness for any reason, even if it was when you were a tiny baby?"

"No, never, Doctor. I know I was a healthy baby. And there's no family history of seizures or epilepsy. I've never been knocked out and I've never fainted. No headaches, or dizziness, or recent changes in my mental function either, Doctor. And I don't drink. I just can't understand what happened. It *really* took me by surprise!"

By now you're examining the fundi and maybe, for a few style points, you're putting the bell of your stethoscope on his temple. After all, those AVMs can be noisy. Today isn't *new-onset seizure day.* That's far too innocent, Doc. Today the agenda is:

What has this man's seizure threshold been like over his lifetime? Is there anything about him that suggests a recent change in the tissue in his head?

Your agenda contains a presenting complaint that has been previewed, digested, and put in the context of the patient's global health and disease status. You can't enter that room without an agenda, with the mindset: *Well, let's see what's going on with the man in Room Three.* You *know* what your opening line is going to be. You know exactly where your physical examination is going to start. And you know how you're going to wind things up. The rest is juggling differential diagnoses, putting a live unique human being into the equation, and having your courage and wits about you if your patient throws you a curve.

Zen Break

You will create for yourself a sacred moment just before you enter the room where your next patient awaits you. You will use the pause with every patient. Neither your staff nor your patient will ever see it. The Zen Break is your secret and incredibly powerful tool. You are standing alone in the hall, patient chart in hand, and the door is closed.

Erase all memories and thoughts of your previous patient, all cares and concerns of the day. Let your mind go blank as you enter a state of mini-meditation. Now you let all you know of the patient on the other side of the door flood you—her words, her physical findings, her studies—all your previous experience with her and all your reconstructions of her illness and her disease.

Now, open her chart and refresh your mind with numerical data and details from the last exam—the little personalizing notes you made about her dog, her daughter's birthday party, and her dislike for Stravinsky. Walk around inside her in your mind.

Picture this patient of yours behind the door. Picture her inside and out, head to toe, rostral to caudal, dorsal to ventral, awake and asleep, in her own world and now in the world of the clinic. You have heard what she has said before and yet you have heard nothing. Think of her as a citizen and then as a specimen and then neither.

Perhaps this is akin to those few seconds when the house lights dim and the conductor steps to the podium. Then he stands and taps his baton. He raises it, and the music comes forth. Now you can enter that examining room.

At first, the Zen Break will strain your mind. It will be a little painful. Breathe in, breathe out. That's the point.

You're preparing for an intense seven minutes of total patient focus that will demand all your energy and a goodly chunk of your brain.

All of a sudden, as if by magic, it's all new, fresh, and clear. Your prejudging thoughts, *I know what she's going to say . . . I've heard it before,* will vanish. And now you're free to entertain new differentials, other approaches, and alternative models of what's going on with her.

How long will you be standing there? At first, about 40 seconds; after a couple of months, about 20. Take as long as it takes, as long as you want. Add a little Tai Chi to the mix. Let your brain recharge an amp or two. Besides, you'll live longer. You deserve it, and your patient does too.

As far as theater is concerned, the Zen Break cranks up your charisma when you *do* open that door. You'll look rested, unhurried, and ready to devote. You show no hint of a furrowed brow and no fuzziness of purpose. All the pages have been flipped. You're the right stuff.

You've seen the haggard doc who's not about to pause for Zen or anything else. She barges in on the patient unprepared, her head buried in the chart. And she's sporting a plus-three frown in full bloom:

"Oh yes, you're the one with the chest x-ray that looked like it might be lung cancer. Was it left or right? I can't remember. I can't seem to locate the film. Anyway, I thought I had the biopsy report right here; it looks like cancer. By the way, you're a smoker, aren't you?"

The poor doc's frazzled, and so is her poor patient, who already wants a second opinion and maybe a new doctor too.

The Zen Break will sharpen and brighten you. The aura of enlightened understanding alone is worth the 20-second investment. And you'll save time too, far more than you can imagine. After six months or so of practice, you'll find yourself floating into that room on undiluted mental energy. And a good pair of shoes.

The Set

The examination room is a stage, and you and the patient are players. As the curtain goes up, that person in the crowd of the waiting area is transformed into a patient, and the figure wearing a white coat suddenly becomes her doctor. Within these few square feet, matters of life and death may get talked over, orifices may be explored, and the soul can be bared. The space is dedicated to the observation of the only central character, your patient.

The room is spotless, the air is fresh, and there are no sounds of the outside world to be heard. Neither cold floor nor instruments will chill your patient. All the furnishings will be essential and none will be cheap or shabby. The decor is a kind of Spartan elegance.

In glancing around the room it is impossible to detect that any other patient has ever been there. There are no x-rays or lab slips or charts belonging to others. There are no used gloves or body fluids in sight, and there is nothing to peek at in the wastebasket. There is no clock. The telephone isn't going to ring, and no pagers are going to beep. For these few moments, devoted exclusively to her visit, the rest of humanity vanishes and time is suspended.

Patients are voyeurs. They will study your examination room or your office for clues about your character, your interests, and your life. Give them what you want them to see. Clear out junk, knickknacks that reflect politics or religion, and photographs of you doing anything but accepting the Nobel Prize in medicine. Thou shalt have no cheap plastic stomach models.

This is the workroom of a skilled technician who has a deep understanding of disease and the human condition.

The tools of your trade and a few carefully arranged diplomas tell a good enough story. Artwork is to be meticulously chosen and displayed with great care. After all, this is the domain of a wise, gifted, and benevolent practitioner of the healing arts who happens, for seven minutes, to be your patient's physician.

Hospitality and Traffic

Hotel and restaurant managers know that success depends on smooth turnover, keeping their guests and patrons in a state of coming and going rather than moving in and homesteading. And when it's done right, there's that marvelous sense of timelessness, of being able to stay as long as you like. Looked at from afar, everyone appears busy and no one rushed.

You, too, are in a certain kind of hospitality enterprise. Your patients leave their homes for a brief adventure in medicine and then return. These are people in motion, and it is essential that you know the patterns of their movements. Study pedestrian traffic in other doctors' clinics, and take notes on the flow of people through malls, airports, fast-food places, and Jiffy Lube. Note where things go wrong, where gridlock occurs, where lines start getting longer. Watch the movement of people with walkers and wheelchairs, crutches and canes. Note how caregivers clutch, cling, and navigate. Sooner or later all these folks are going to wind up in your clinic.

In a perfect world your patient wakes up, takes a shower, shows up for her appointment, gets her doctoring done, and leaves your clinic promptly to return to her world of better things to do. She has arrived on time and she will leave on time. She has no interest in lingering in your waiting room. She moves like a gazelle, wears no clothing that can't be removed in one minute, and carries no shopping bags, umbrellas, or luggage—only a small purse that she doesn't leave behind. Her questions and your answers are succinct. She'll perform as well at her next visit too. And you can dream.

Unless you're running a skin clinic for super models, your office is going to be laid out to handle a few nitty-gritty scenarios that will pop up daily. What if we add forty years, Parkinson's, two cataracts, and an ejection fraction of ten? Think traffic flow. Get out your drawing board and start planning where you're going to put your furniture, your examining tables, and your waiting area. Study other clinics, good and bad. Walk yourself through the challenging scenarios—psychosis, quadriplegia, hip fracture, the morbid obesity. Share with your staff. Then rip out a wall or two and start thumbing through equipment catalogs. And while your waiting room is on your mind, subscribe to the most wonderful magazines you can think of. Updating and upgrading your clinic will *always* have priority over redecorating at home. That new kitchen can wait.

Concentrate on the basics of people in motion from their worlds to your clinic and back. How is your patient going to get there? How is he going to move from waiting room to examining room? What about disrobing, gowns, getting up on the table? And what about making it back to the reception room and out the front door? Add to this shopping bags, nursing newborn twins, a dog, and a spouse who's so sick she should be in an ER.

The next time you're in a great hotel or even a good one, make some notes for yourself. How was your arrival handled? What's going on in the lobby? Notice how the front desk was expecting you. How is your trip from the lobby to your room choreographed? Notice how your room immediately becomes your second home. No one was ever in there before. And what about soundproofing from traffic in the hallway and grunts and groans in the next room, the little comfort goodies, and the sense of security?

It's your hotel, doctor. Set the tone, the tempo, and the mood to suit you and your staff. Think ergonomics, and make the decor as comfortable and elegant as you can. This is where you spend your working life.

"How far away do you live?"

"About a hundred miles, Doctor."

"How long does it take you to get here?"

"About three hours, depends on traffic. Martha, my social worker, calls the van driver early in the week. They have a special lift for my wheelchair. He usually has to pick up five or six other passengers and drop them off at the hospital and the other clinics. This is the last stop on his route. I have to wear an extra Attends, like today."

What are you going to do in the next seven minutes, Doctor? What are you going to do that's going to be worth all that effort? It is essential that you master the skill of imagining your patient going through the intricate moves of her daily life. Think of yourself as a surveillance camera monitoring the twitches, breaths, leg-crossings, and bathroom trips of her day. See her getting ready for that van. Then fast forward to imagine how you're going to get her in the stirrups, how that prescription is going to get filled, how the insulin is going to get drawn up.

"Mrs. Putamen is going to be rolling in in about five minutes. Let's put her in Room One as soon as she gets here. She likes it warm in there. It might take three of us to get her up in the stirrups. Let me know as soon as she arrives and I'll come out and give you a hand. It's her grandson's birthday. Let her know we remembered. Find out if we can help her with the prescriptions. She'll need help with the insulin. I'll talk to the pharmacist. Remember, she has those cataracts that haven't been taken care of yet. And she'll need some help getting back in the van. By the way, as soon as Mr. Baipole arrives, get him in Room Two and I'll come in *immediately*. We can take care of the paperwork while he's in there. We all remember what happened with him in the waiting room last month!"

It's your hotel, Doctor. Maybe not the Ritz, but still yours.

Crew

You and your staff are equals. Every day you all plunge into the fluxus of getting the sick in and out of your clinic in an atmosphere of elegance, kindness, and efficiency. It's a seamless, classless enterprise. Sure you're the boss, but that's trivial.

Pay everyone well. Make the clinic delightful to work in, a space where complaints are unknown. Give all of you a vacation when the communal energy looks like it's about to wane. Buy thoughtful gifts, and in every way be generous.

If for one picosecond any member of your staff gives anything less than her best, fire her. Stat.

Narcissus

Your practice of medicine is not about you. Your patient was not created or morphed in your image. She happens to be in your clinic today by a quirk of fate. It is a though you were walking through a rain forest and a strange new creature plopped on your head. So don't take it personally if she appears to be a little unreasonable. It isn't your doing.

There are two people in that examining room of yours. All the attention, every millimole of it, is directed toward the patient. There is no room for talking about you, dear doctor. Not one word. That's why the magic works.

Watch your transference! That's everything flying through the air of the examining room that doesn't have a deeply rational quality. The strength of your relationship with the patient is your knowledge and your experience with human disease. She is not your friend, your enemy, or your kin. And you are not a best-friend's-shoulder-to-cry-on, nor a priest, nor a talk show host. Or guest. Neither are you a guidance counselor, advice columnist, or whipping boy.

Amateur psychiatry is dangerous. Any warm and fuzzy feeling between doctor and patient deserves a good hard look. The great physicians are those who have spent time—a lot of time—examining and coming to terms with their feelings about their patients. Pay attention to your patients' appearances in your dreams. Critique the feelings and fantasies that you bring to *every* clinic visit with *every* patient. They are paying for objectivity—not for pity, sentimentality, contempt, or romantic love. If you wake up with a warp in your transference, take the day off.

The visit is the patient's time, not an opportunity to talk about your Ferrari or your gifted and beautiful children or your mountain climbing. Channel your entire glorious ego into an engrossing study of the human being sitting before you. Humility saves time and frees energy for practicing medicine. By resisting the temptation to inject personal anecdotes, you concentrate the patient's interests on introspection and accurate self-description.

The two of you are looking at his dizziness. You aren't comparing dizziness stories over our lifetimes:

"Doctor, have you ever been so drunk you felt the room spin?"

Not batting an eyelash, and with a kind smile and the eye contact of a hawk, you reply, "Tell me what that's like and how it compares to your recent dizziness."

When asked next, "Doctor, haven't you ever had a headache?," you draw your chair a bit closer, smiling again, and reply, "I'm curious why you asked." It's not that the physician is above human frailty and the flotsam and jetsam of living in the world, but this doctor's life, at the moment, is concentrated entirely on the patient.

It is very easy to make patients love you and think you're great. Send out just the faintest bat squeak of Eros and you have a crush on your hands. You do not *need* your patients' love, just as you don't *need* their admiration and kind remarks. Be loved elsewhere. Save your confidences and passion for your partner, your family, your dear friends, and your dog.

Patients bring us gifts from time to time. Accept them with kindness and gracious courtesy, but look at the act of giving, too, as a part of the transference. We are in a profession that deals with caring and nurturing, with an intense focus on the suffering part of the human condition. These matters are inherently invested with great passion. Be sublime, be vigilant, and be circumspect.

Let your patients find out how wonderful you are through their improved health and well-being. Don't fall into the trap of believing "*My patients need me.*" They don't. They need their health and their autonomy. That's good enough. If you still need to be seen as something special, keep in mind that creating an aura of mystery about you invokes considerable elegance. The true identity of the superhero eludes the patients of Gotham.

Being a doctor doesn't mean you can get away with saying, *"You're going to do this because I said so."* You have no divine powers, no omniscience, and no license to proclaim off-the-cuff insults like "I don't think there's anything wrong with you." Never patronize, never condescend, and never argue.

Physicians think they're bright, but you'll have patients far more intelligent than you who simply don't have your kind of training. Once in a while you'll have a doctor as a patient. He'll give you a little lesson in the nature of demystification and the chilling reality that you're just another human being who, like him, went to an expensive trade school.

Everyone dies—you and every one of your patients. Fate, disease, and doctors take the rap. You're in good company, up there with the megaforces of human destiny. Physicians, if we do nothing else, bear witness to the human condition. We make up the rules of disease and its treatment on our watch, and before we know it we're swallowed up in history. Once in a while, though, you'll hear a colleague getting rhapsodic in thinking that he's made some small difference in the lives of the folks he's treated. Nonsense—just narcissism in sentimental clothing.

Be honest, be scholarly, and be kind to your patients. Avoid developing a taste for being worshipped. You aren't Elvis.

Chores

Alas! You've figured out by now that most of medical practice has to do with the clinical equivalents of putting clothes in the dryer, calling the plumber, and picking up a few things at the market. Not to mention vacuuming and figuring out where you put that Phillips screwdriver. Insurance forms, handicapped parking applications, back-to-work slips, and prescription refills can take away from the excitement and theme of the visit if you let them. To prevent this, deliver the results of lab results and tests before moving on. This will solve the problem of your patient looking so preoccupied while you're finishing up what you think is a perfectly marvelous seven-minute exam, only to ask, "Doc, what did my tests show?" Those results were all she wanted today, the only reason she kept the appointment. Whatever other doctoring you thought you were doing was wasted.

Every clinic visit has a beginning, middle, and end. The beginning lines are always yours, and they establish the theme of the day. The middle four or five minutes are the rolled-up-sleeves segment that combines Socratic commentary with hammer-and-tongs examination. The end is your summing-up, patient-removal, and paving the way for the next visit.

Chores belong at the beginning. Anywhere else they detract from the purpose of the visit, interrupt the flow, and deflate the sense of conclusion. Sometimes all your patient wants is to get chores out of the way:

"Doc, I know this is a lot to fill out, but I have to have it for my job. They won't let me go back to work without it."

So take care of it right now. Until proven otherwise, an envelope is a chore. Take care of it first and do your doctoring with whatever time is left over:

"I notice you have some papers with you. Are they something we need to take care of?"

Sometimes there's just that blank look when you walk in the door—that look that tells you that no doctoring is going to get done until you do the housekeeping:

"Is there something we need to be taking care of this morning? You look like you've got something on your mind. Tell me . . ."

"That prescription you gave me—the pharmacist told me it cost a hundred dollars. I don't have a hundred dollars, and my insurance doesn't cover it."

"Let me write for something else, and I'll have Martha call over and find out what it costs. Is that all right?"

Sometimes chores are medical touchups. Your patient with Bell's palsy wants to know only one thing: *Is it a stroke?* You, on the other hand, have launched into a lecture on the pathophysiology of the facial nerve in which she has zero interest. "By the way, this is not a stroke," delivered *immediately* after your initial examination would have done the trick. *"Thanks, doctor, that's really all I wanted to know."* Now you're free to talk about corneal abrasions, prednisone, and prognosis. Get your chores out of the way and then you can play, Doctor.

The Touch

Every visit includes touch. You can talk for an hour with impassioned empathy, and your patient will go away thinking you're probably a nice person and you seemed to be listening—but you didn't do anything. Touch every patient on every visit. It doesn't matter where. You can feel the neck, poke around in the belly, or put a stethoscope in the popliteal fossa or a tuning fork on the iliac crest if you like. Touch and talk while you're focussing the dialog on the body part in hand:

"As I remember *(making a dent in the plus-four tibial edema)* you were taking 80 milligrams of Lasix twice a day."

While you're saying this, gently feel the jugular vein, listen to the chest, and take the radial pulse: "Are you still having to pause half-way up the stairs to your bedroom?"

By now, with a comforting arm around the shoulder, you can narrow your questioning to the specifics of chest pain, dyspnea, and medication tolerance. You've physically fused diagnosis with therapy, and you've paved the way for speedy exit.

Do a touch even if your patient has stopped by for a 90-second pill refill. Take that pulse. Brief though it may be, you've completed a real physical exam, and you can write a solid miniature progress note to go along with it. *Refill metoprolol. Tolerated well. No chest pain since last visit. Pulse 60 and regular.* So, maybe another ten seconds for entering the note?

If a new complaint crops up in the midst of today's visit, immediately get your hands on some part of the anatomy that at least symbolically relates to the symptom. "I forgot to tell you, Doc—I've been feeling real dizzy lately," may be handled as follows: Reach over, put your hand behind the neck, and gently tilt the head:

"Are you dizzy now?"

Put on a cuff and check the pressure—have her stand up and check it again. Then *you* stand up. And keep moving.

"Let's go out in the hall and take a look at your walking."

Then bend him over and stand him back up.

"Dizzy now?"

Keep your hands on your patient for that reassuring sense of stability, and without missing a beat, carry on with your stage directing:

"Let me see you walk a little with your eyes closed."

Continue to encourage maximal effort, to reassure that he won't collapse, and to watch for that elusive dizziness to emerge. If you find it useful to have your patient hyperventilate or to perform some variation on a theme of Valsalva, then keep your fingers on the radial pulse or maybe somewhere on the head or neck during the exercise. Palpation is comforting and gives the impression that you're monitoring something. At this point you can inject whatever questions you like. You'll find that the answers you get in the midst of all these gymnastics are far more relevant and precise than what you'd obtain with the two of you seated on either side of an oak desk.

If your patient starts talking about itching teeth, then reach *immediately* for a tongue blade and get inside that mouth. When he realizes that you're probing for a real mass, and you look like you might actually *find* something, he'll be far more accepting of the ultimate diagnosis. *"He didn't seem to believe what I was saying"* most often gets muttered when the physical examination is half-hearted or just wasn't done.

The exam should always mean something to you or to your patient. Perform every examination on every visit with the true intent of *finding* something or with the equally sincere intent of letting the patient know you're on the case. There should be no other reason. Going through the motions of an apathetic exam because "that's the way they taught us we have to do it" portrays an indifference that your patient will immediately pick up. You may not think you're likely to find a thyroid nodule by palpating the neck today, but if you poke around with sincerity, enthusiasm, and the spirit of a truffle-sniffing pig, your patient will honor the pursuit.

The entire exam may be quite brief, a matter of seconds—flipping over an eyelid, a little pressure on a fingernail, a pinch, or 60 long seconds of dedicated pulse taking. It is the act of touching, with purpose and intelligence flowing through the finger, that makes Michaelangelo's fresco of God and Adam so compelling. If you do it right, your patient will leave your office feeling a bit revitalized, believing you know more and understand more about her. You have touched her life.

Words and Organs

In the grand scheme of history, medicine is at its best when doctors are doing something else besides talking to patients—like cutting and pasting, inoculating, and spraying swamps with insecticides. Second best is the doctor snuggled up with her own private language, talking into a machine in the privacy of a comfy office, spewing out phrases like *immunocytologic dissociation, anaplastic oligodendroglioma,* or *endothelial integrity.* It's jargon like this that got us seduced into thinking that medicine was *scientific* and that somehow, with a clever trick or wave of a fiberoptic wand, we were going to create a histopathological correlate to the poetry that comes out of our patients' mouths.

It all falls apart, though, when Ms. Hyster serves up her presenting complaint: "It feels like an octopus is sucking my brains out." We're forever searching for something that splashes when we drop it in formalin. So, do we flip to the index of *Cecil's* or *Harrison's* and start searching for Cephalopoda? And pray for a subheading under partial vacuums?

Mathematicians and physicists are the most amused by all this. After all, they have it the easiest, playing their game with the very symbols and standards for proof they created. We physicians are stuck dealing with a soft, warm, moist machine that we didn't design. It talks, but we find out fast that its speech circuits don't match up with its anatomy, let alone telling us in any consistent pattern what's *really* happening when it breaks down.

There are ways of getting around the word-illness problem of course. Veterinarians, with the exception of Dr.

Dolittle, practice fine face-to-face medicine without any doctor-patient dialog at all. And the dermatologist knows that no matter what her patient says, the disease is out there in full view. Take a peek, punch that skin, and slap on one of those great words like *serpiginous* and a steroid cream. Word flow like "It feels like little worms crawling around under there" may add some fun to the visit, but it doesn't stand in the way of getting things done. Radiology is even better, and pathology the best. How exhilarating to know *what I say is always the truth, on my terms, in my own words, and I've never had a conversation with a patient.*

There is a sort of hybrid post-modern approach—reducing the complaint to a course of action without pausing to wonder about linguistic subtleties. A few key words serve to trigger the procedure. "Every time I eat calf's liver I get nauseated" buys the patient an EGD. And, further down, "Every time I eat garbanzos I get gas" schedules a colonoscopy. No further questions and no critique of the poetry enter into the scheme. Thus our octopus gets an MRI of the head, and any use of the word "back" gets an MRI of the territory.

Why in the world, then, do you want to have a dialog with your patient, and what do you want the exchange to do for you? Words are the realm of the human, the expression of being alive in the world, the I and the Thou of it all. Words falling on your ears are the patient's illness. Your modeling of them, enhanced with an examination and a few labs, becomes the disease. *That* part is your doing. While illness is personal gut-spilling, disease is ultimately public domain. We want to tap into that private world because we want the patient's perspective and we want a transference that will be helpful in getting our job done.

The universal problem with language in the clinic is the signal-to-noise ratio. We listen to hours of verbal fillers and shopworn similes. *It feels like a tight band. . . . It feels like my stomach is being blown up like a balloon. . . . It feels like I'm walking on basketballs.* Is there a remedy?

You can start by eliminating a lot of noise. Gossip, politics, religion, scenes from the wonderful doctor's life, all get trashed. Doctors talk too much. If you're breezy and sloppy in your language, your dear patient will follow suit. Being long-winded tires you both and detracts from your mystique.

Gently and firmly expect and demand precision:

"I don't have a clear idea of what you mean by *fuzzy headed.*"

"You know, Doc, kind of fuzzy, kind of foggy, kinda in a haze. . . ."

"I really *don't.* Why not give me an example?"

At this point you move closer, perhaps 3 or 4 inches, and put your palm on his forehead, rocking it almost imperceptibly.

"Like time has stopped. I can keep moving and I'm sort of aware of what's going on, but I can't talk. Like the way you feel just as you're falling asleep."

This 45-second interaction is solid gold. It's personalized, enhances the nature of the symptom through physical contact, and invites trust. It may not have given you an immediate diagnosis, but it put both of you where you need to be, in the land of the brain. No emergency colonoscopy at any rate.

Train your patients to function as journalists, bringing you descriptions of the action that goes with the feeling:

"It was throbbing so bad."

"What did you do?"

"I just stood there and waited for it to pass"

"Did you close your eyes? Did you stagger? Could you have kept walking if you'd had too?"

You know that your technique is working when you can see your patient having one of her events in your mind's eye.

"Could you feel yourself falling?"

"Yes, but I'd lost my sight. It was completely grayed out. But I could feel my knees buckling."

"And when you came to, what was the first thing you saw?"

"I couldn't have been out for more than five seconds. I knew where I was. I was looking up at Diane, who was bending down to help me up."

It's as though you're there on the street with a video camera catching every detail of the action. When the critical moment arrives, you move in for the close-up, keeping your focus sharp and your wits about you.

Words aren't objects, and they aren't truth or disease. Repeat this to yourself on your way to the clinic. Words, though, are the essence of the narrative-bound disorders, and some very graphic ones at that. About once a year we see a couple who remind us of how easily we can make the fatal erroneous leap from language to tissue:

"Tell me about the mass in your neck."

"Every morning about 5 o'clock it swells up right here."

"Show me."

Mr. Massa gestures with his palm, making a circular movement as though smoothing out a snowball. His wife nods in agreement:

"That's right, Doctor. I can feel it too, just like he said."

"And it's real hard and tight. I can feel the pressure in there, and it's sore—real sore. After about half an hour it goes down and you wouldn't know it had been there. Next morning that lump's right back, about the size of a small grapefruit. You could set your watch by it."

Is your reality testing being tested? No, dear doctor, only your fundamentalist belief in the truth-telling property of language. This is the same word-craft that brought us *Hamlet*, *Dracula*, cold fusion, and the Loch Ness monster. What we learn from our phantom-tumor vignette, namely that words are words and tissue is tissue, will serve us well when we're dealing with the more common narratives of chronic fatigue, fibromyalgia, and attention deficit disorder. *Give me your motor stuff. Give me something I can picture. Give me a right-brain script.*

To stay in shape, flip through an issue of *Nature* now and then. Or one of the physics or microbiology journals if the mood strikes you. There isn't a "you know" or a "creepy crawly queasy feeling" between any of *those* covers, is there? Later, with a little inspired rigor, you might demystify some of your patient's laments:

"How long do they last?"

"Not too long, Doc."

"Seconds? Less than a minute?"

"Maybe 20 seconds. Never more than half a minute."

"Has even one of them lasted less than ten seconds?"

"No. Never."

All this sounds nit-picky and obsessive, but there's a method in this madness of asking for, in fact demanding, precision. After a few visits your patient will learn that you won't take "Oh, I don't know. Not very often I guess. . ." as an answer. He may become less vague about the rest of his dealings with you, too.

Show and Tell

Get specific about the boundaries of the symptom during that first minute of the examination. Your staff will let you know ahead of time if a gown and chaperone are going to be needed as you gear up for your adventure in visceral cartography.

"Show me with one finger where the pain starts and where it goes from there."

Mr. Vaag moves his hand through the air as though shooing a fly, at best referring to something going on below the torso.

"With one finger—trace it for me."

Now the Vaag is rubbing his thigh with his palm.

"Where does it start? Does it go over here? Does it travel up or down?"

You have your finger on the thigh, doing some drawing of your own and asking for Vaag's confirmation or revision of the sketch. By now he's using *one* finger, and correcting you, too.

Use the patient's body as a blackboard. Or as a lump of modeling clay. Where he touches, you touch. Where he points, you palpate. Where he cups his hand, you plop down your stethoscope. Don't sit back while the patient gestures. Get right in the thick of him. It doesn't hurt to percuss a little if the mood strikes you. Stay in the area, and linger there with your fingers and tools long enough to get in a couple of questions about frequency, duration, and associated symptoms. Then, when you sit back two or three minutes from now and put together an explanatory model, it will have a visceral echo for your patient. Think chiropractor, phrenologist, and masseuse—all practitioners of the concentrated touch.

The ambiguity of the word "feel" can be used to great advantage:

"It feels like the bottom of my foot's on fire."

"Let's take a look at it. Let me feel it. Here?"

"You've got your hand right on it, Doctor! Can you feel it too?" *Of course I can—maybe not what you're feeling, but that's OK. We're in this together.*

Thinking quickly, you pull out a tuning fork, twang it, and put it on his big toe:

"Feel this? Tell me when it stops vibrating. . . ."

During all this you've kept your own fingers on his toes or sole, touching and supporting the foot while the tuning fork buzzes. Borrow from the foot massage experts. Let energy flow through your fingertips. You've just directed a tiny multimedia production.

"Show and Tell" can be adapted to give substance to dynamic body-in-motion complaints. "I feel dizzy when I stand up" deserves palpating and tracking the act of standing up. In addition to doing blood pressure cuff orthostatics, palpate a selection of pulses sitting and standing. Put your stethoscope on a carotid and your palm on the occiput while he stands. *My doctor is right there when it's happening!* Well, sort of. . . .

If a body part is offered, you are obligated to palpate it. It's as absolute as a hand offered in greeting. You've completed the most marvelous gem of an examination, with a perfect summing up and effective plans for a future visit, but just as your patient reaches the door she turns around and says: "Oh, by the way, Doctor, I've been having this pain in my ear." Unless you get out your otoscope and look inside, you've done *nothing*, and the entire rest of the exam goes up in smoke.

Once in a while when you ask a patient to do something, he gets it wrong. You've asked him to hold up the right hand and he gives you the left. Or you ask him to open his mouth and he sticks out his tongue. Examine both hands, the one offered first, then the one you wanted. Look at that tongue and nod. *My doctor is thorough and patient and never makes me feel stupid. I can show her anything.* Isn't this the trust and confidence you've been cultivating all along, Doctor?

The Eye

The eye is still the window of the soul, even in the era of magnetic resonance imaging. Examining the eye, particularly when the complaint of the day is tingling in the umbilicus, is always perceived as fine doctoring. The message is: "I can peer into your inner self, into your brain and mind." And so you can. Why not, though, let your patient know what you're up to?

"The blood vessels in your retina show some of the changes we see with diabetes. The retina itself looks good, and so does the optic nerve. Let's take a look at the other side."

"You can actually see all *that*, Doc?"

The mystique of the darkened room, and the fact that you're *not* an eye doctor can work to your advantage.

In a way, the ophthalmoscope is akin to the polygraph. "Does anyone in your family have high blood pressure?" you ask, with the lights dimmed and the instrument beaming right into your patient's memory and soul. Metaphors abound: *"She can see through me. She's getting into my head."* Yes.

You have been penetrating and meticulous. The entire operation took you no more than thirty seconds. And it was far more sublime than a digital rectal exam.

Am I Interrupting You?

"I understand you had a fainting spell? Would you like to tell me about it?"

"Well, as you know, Doctor, we've been married 50 years—met at a high school basketball game, and Bill was wearing the funniest hat I'd ever seen. Well, the kids—we've got six scattered all over the country—and the grandkids decided to give us a surprise anniversary party. You just can't imagine! The loveliest cake—you know, those little rosettes like years ago, and real hand-dipped candles, little bitty ones, real beeswax. I don't know how they did it."

Nor do I, Mrs. Logree. And how in the world can I bring myself to flip back to the fainting-spell channel and risk hurting your dear feelings? Should I cancel the rest of today's clinic and let the party unfold? Did you bring any pictures?

We are taught that interrupting is rude and that we are to begin the dissection of the presenting complaint with broad strokes, generalities, and open-ended questions. Wrong. You are a drama coach, a film director, and a personal trainer for the art of effective history-giving. You are coaxing and bringing out the narrative—delivering it by Cesarean section if necessary. If this role doesn't suit you, then think of yourself, machete in hand, slashing through vines and underbrush in your quest of the lost city. Think archeologist on a dig, kneeling down in the sand with a trowel and camel hair brush, unearthing and bringing to light the buried artifacts of forgotten lives.

Just as it is the musician's challenge to keep the music afloat, to keep the harmonic structure off the ground, so is it your job to keep the disease-illness axis balanced and moving toward resolution. Radio interviewers know that there can be no empty airtime. You must continually be anticipating the next question and answer, remaining a step ahead of your patient's immediate response. Begin with physical and visceral specifics, making it clear that you're pursuing accuracy, graphic detail, and a richly rendered reconstruction of your patient's valued memory of her experience. You know what you *wanted* to say:

"Mrs. Logree, you're the only one in this room who can shed some light on what happened, the only one who knows what that felt like, and what your body was doing at the moment. Tell me about it. Where were you standing? What time was it? What did your daughter Helen say you looked like?"

Shall we start over? You have decided beforehand that the business of the day is *figuring out the nature of her spell* and relating it to her disease trends to date. Entering the room, you remain standing, and reach out to gently palpate her radial pulse, placing a couple of your other fingers on her temple.

"I understand you passed out. Could you feel yourself falling to the ground?"

"Like I told the nurse, we were at the most wonderful surprise party. . . ."

"Stand up for a moment. There—are you lightheaded?"

"A little."

"Did you feel like *this* just before you passed out?"

"No."

"What time was it?"

"About ten thirty."

"Had you had any breakfast?"

"No."

"Had you taken your insulin?"

"Yes, at around six."

"What about your Lasix and atenolol?"

"Yes, and I was on my way to the bathroom?"

"To urinate?"

"Yes, we'd been in the car all morning. You see we were running late and . . ."

"When you got out of the car did you feel lightheaded?"

"Well, I guess, but we had her teddy bear in the . . ."

"So you got out of the car with the teddy bear? Then what happened?"

"We walked over to the picnic table. My knee was bothering me."

"And that was about how far from where you parked?"

By now, and this has taken about 90 seconds, Mrs. Logree's got the idea. You aren't being rude at all—you're helping her put it all together. In order for this to work, your eye contact has to be perfect, and you're going to have your hands on some body part. Your dialog will include remnants of Mrs. L's previous words, indicating that you are a fine and fascinated listener. You're going from specific to even more specific, and the flattery of your being absolutely *intrigued* with what happened at the party will get you where you want to go. Let the non-sequiturs fall where they may. Think cross-examination. Take your ophthalmoscope and dim the lights:

"So how old were you the first time you fainted? How many times have you passed out in your whole life, or been unconscious for any reason at all? Is there anybody else in the family with spells?"

"Well, the first time I ever passed out was when I was twelve, around my first period, and mom took me to the doctor because I was having headaches. The nurse was taking some blood and I looked down and saw the needle and out I went."

"Have all your spells been like that first one?"

Here you're appealing to Mrs. L's intellect, to her powers of self-analysis. *You're a bright woman, Mrs. Logree—let's see if you can come up with a diagnosis.*

None of this is going to work if you're sitting five feet away with your arms crossed. Nor is it going to work if you're thumbing through her medical record or doing a lot of patronizing nodding and umhumming. You're not bored—you're engrossed. You're on the edge of your seat. You want *more*!

"What's the lowest blood sugar reading you've had in the past year?"

"Forty—that I know of."

"And how did you feel with a blood sugar of 40?"

"Kind of woozy"

"Was the wooziness anything like how you felt before you passed out?"

"Pretty much the same."

Just as one of the cardinal principles of cross-examination is don't cross-examine, so is it with history-taking. Ideally the need for interruption won't come up. If you begin with a question that is perfectly attuned to your patient's experience, reflecting your intimate knowledge of her past history, you'll be rewarded in kind. And, with only a few snips of your pruning shears here and there, you're *done*.

Cut to the Chase

In the course of your career, you may run into half a dozen almost perfect patients. They communicate with you as though by telepathy, have a realistic sense of their health and disease, and show up on time. They know the quirks and limitations of the current state of the healing art, and they have a sense of humor about the whole health-care sphere. Maybe they're angels.

With these dear hearts you may risk the dangerous questions: "How are you feeling? How have you been getting along since I last saw you? How are you?"
But *only* with them. Your daily work simply can't tolerate inviting disaster with phrases like: "And how may I be of help to you?" You aren't a telemarketer, and you're not running a burger joint.

The words coming out of your mouth when you enter that room have already been trimmed down to the ultra-specific:

"Let's take a look at that ear of yours—and the other one for comparison. You've been having that drainage for a week? When you had that ear infection a year ago, I believe it responded to Cipro. Let's put you back on it for ten days."

About thirty seconds have elapsed, and you're already past the wax staring right at the tympanic membrane. To deliver this punch you've skimmed the chart and been clued in by your receptionist that it's ear day—*right* ear day, in fact. Three minutes ago you actually saw yourself in your mind's eye reaching for the otoscope and tongue blade, peeking in ear and mouth, palpating the neck, and writing a prescription.

In the less-than-extreme world the opening might have been: "What seems to be the problem today?" Then, with a let-me-get-myself-up-to-speed look on your face: "Oh, yes, your ear. Tell me about your ear. Is it the left or the right? Have you ever had ear problems before? As far as you know are you allergic to any antibiotics? So tell me, how long have you been having this drainage?"

"Well, Doctor, when I was a kid I used to have a lot of ear infections and mom took me to the doctor all the time, and he talked about putting tubes in my ears. Antibiotics, well, let me think. I seem to remember once that I had a rash from, was it ampicillin? But that was years ago."

We recall those painful and humiliating ten-page history and physical write-ups from medical school days. They were all wrong, not only because they had no relevance in the real world but because we lost the essence of what was going on with the patient in a forest of system review. And then came our coup de grace, a mindless head-to-toe groping of irrelevant body parts.

Your patient knew it too. He may have patiently gone along with the whole thing and submitted to the rectal exam when all he wanted was something for his sinus infection. But he never thought you were doing medicine. There may have been a lot of detail, but no priorities—a lot of telling but no true showing. We simply weren't taught how to grab onto that symptom and, as though riding a bronco, just refuse to let go.

It doesn't matter what opening move you choose as long as it captures the essence of your patient's illness. You are limited to nothing. You may choose to deal with a single phrase—breathlessness, pallor, a wobbly gait. You may walk in the door with the differential diagnosis of *new-onset jaundice in 30-year-old females* running through your head as if it was a song. You may decide, on some capricious hunch, to start with a certain body region—a hand perhaps.

"You've been having some tingling in the fingers? Which ones? Show me. When I tap right *here* what happens?"

If you want to forfeit your first move and let your patient start with "I have something to tell you, Doc," know from the beginning that you'll have some catching up to do. With your stethoscope in your ears, pull up a chair and start listening to something. Anything. Then, pulling back one earpiece: "I'm listening. When was that?"

Then listen for the phrase that will set the tone for the visit: "I've been having these spells where I just black out for a few seconds."

Now you can close in. Do the heart valves and do the carotids since you're in the neighborhood—but from this point on it's brain day—and therefore calvarium and eyes.

Be prepared, in the blink of an eye, to abandon the plan you'd sketched out so carefully but a moment ago. You walk into the room and notice your patient has changed dramatically since the last visit. There's no particular complaint and no heads up from Joyce, except "Mr. Cancro doesn't look so good today. He just looks different." The new jaundice, cachexia, cyanosis, the visage of overwhelming depression, stare you in the face the moment you walk in.

"Mr. Cancro, that CT of your abdomen was normal. But I can see you've lost a lot of weight since last month. Looks like more than twenty pounds.

"Closer to thirty, Doc."

"Tell me about your appetite. What did you eat yesterday?" Your plan was a road map. All of a sudden you've run into a detour. Let the detour become an adventure in itself, a plunging into uncharted pathology. Your well-planned agenda, for once, can wait.

Rules and Decisions

Rules are much easier to work with than decisions. Jiffy Lube and restaurants with numbers on their menus know this well. *I'd like the oil changed and a number three and a side order of eleven please.* No art, no abstraction, no analysis.

Pilots, despite their apparent passion for excitement, truly prefer a plane to run on automatic whenever possible. As the technology has gained complexity, what was once a series of learned, conscious, occasionally sweaty actions has become etchings on silicon. So is it with medicine.

Chest pain gets the serial enzymes and EKGs and the nitro drip. The drop of blood on the toilet paper gets guaic cards and the scope. Weight loss and cough go to CT of the chest and a bronchoscopy. While rules may be lousy for delving into the mystique of the individual patient, they're great for pathology-in-populations, for tracking and managing diseases with predictable courses.

Take the top 30 chronic disease scenarios you find yourself reliving, create your own algorithms for them, and have the templates run by your staff. Whenever you find yourself tempted to use the word "routine," make the action involved into a new flow sheet. When you hear yourself spouting out boilerplate explanations and instructions, or when you start repeating words and phrases over and over, stop and re-write your script. This is algorithmic stuff—turn it over to your crew.

Use that brilliant and superbly trained mind of yours for weighing differential diagnoses, listening to your patient's metaphors, personalizing your tender loving care. You are being paid to diagnose and decide on treatment, to analyze your patient's symptoms in the context of her disease—to think *medically* about her. Leave the rest to the autopilot.

Be willing to abandon your templates on super-short notice—the moment you find yourself talking about your patient's view of disease, about his autonomy:

"I know that it's commonplace for people with my kind of blockage to have bypass surgery, doctor. But I just don't want it, and I don't think I want one of those angioplasties either."

This is decision material, not a time for rules. For the next 4 minutes your staff can be busy with someone else.

"I think another major surgery would be too much of a risk right now. I don't have to tell you that, after what you've been through these past six months. Why don't we keep you on the same medications for the time being? If you keep having TIAs, then we can reconsider."

Three minutes from now you can return him to the world of algorithms, to the arms of your loyal staff who can plug him back into lipid, blood pressure, and glucose monitoring—the rule-based aspects of his health. In the meantime he needs his doctor. Do your little vascular exam with heavy emphasis on the neck and heart. Listen to his feelings about surgery in general and about carotid surgery in particular. Mention a few highlights of his past post-op experiences and give him some statistics to mull over. Over and out.

Suffering favors decisions, while stable disease and health favor rules. Make it clear that it is your patient's *disease* you've been tracking with rules, not him, not that unique and special Mr. Cordae:

"You've had a heart attack. I've looked at your angiogram and your EKGs. Your brother Stan and your dad both had heart attacks around the same age, as I remember. If we look at what's happened to you as a blockage of your left anterior descending artery *(pointing to diagram)*, then there are several options."

Here you can shift almost seamlessly to rules, from the individual to the general, from *you my dear patient* to *people with coronary artery disease.* Are you applying a rule or making a decision? Why one and what if the other? Keep an eye on how much of what you're doing today is doctoring and how much of it is straight out of a cookbook.

Satisfaction

A striking feature of mainstream entertainment and fast-food franchises is the overt goal of "pleasing". We are herded in and out of the multiplex having "been to the movies" or, even worse, "feeling good." We are made to leave McDonald's no longer hungry.

But the great chefs and great filmmakers don't really care about whether the public likes their creations or not. What they create has its own value. The question of whether or not the consumer is "right" or not doesn't enter into the picture. So is it with doctoring, dear and glorious physician.

Our job is not to please patients, nor is it—much of the time—to give them what they want. A stiff round of chemotherapy is not a double cheeseburger and a large order of fries. The amputation of a gangrenous foot is not the *Sound of Music*. We survive in our bizarre craft because we provide a respite from the malevolence of the world, a space to let the body show off its frailty. Ours is a safe house for wayward viscera. We win a few and lose a few.

Going to the doctor is akin to a trip to a good library or museum. *If all goes well, dear patient, you'll leave here with a sense of clarity, having had a part of you better defined. You may not like what I find or what I have to say. I may not be able to give you what you want. If you do come back I'll greet you with benevolence, as always. I'm your doctor—no more and no less.*

Expand That Normal

When we started practicing, all those patients had an acute feel to them—simply because they were new to us, because we saw our own observations of their disease as points on the timelines of their lives. We'd never seen the actual patient, nor had we seen how textbook pathologies behaved in the real world. Once a few physical findings were pointed out, the urgency of doing something about the patient's condition became monumental: *Something is terribly wrong and needs my fixing. Right now.*

Those of us who figured out the acute-chronic axis and confronted the cold facts of the curable-incurable early on took the road to surgery. Those whose awakening and disenchantment came even earlier went for radiology and pathology. That left the rest of us.

How long did it take us to realize that it's *normal* for a chronic lunger with advanced heart failure to be out of breath, bloated, dusky, tired, and miserable every minute of his day—not to mention waking up gasping in the middle of the night? After maybe twenty "How are you feeling?" "Terrible, just can't catch my breath" dialogs, we started revising our opening lines:

"Let's take a listen to your chest. Still sleeping on three pillows? Still passing out when you get up too fast? Still unable to keep your shoes on at the end of the day? The last time I saw you, you were able to walk about twenty feet without stopping to catch your breath. Has that changed in the past month?"

"Yes, yes, yes, and about the same—about twenty feet, Doctor." *That's your baseline, that's normal for you. You're normal.*

It takes a year or so to be completely comfortable with shifting the bell curve for wellness over a standard deviation or so. When you're able to take the leap, though, your work with the patient is so much more serene. You're no longer feeling as though your encounters are a matter of going from crisis to crisis.

It's *normal* for your vasculopath to have vasculopathy everywhere. Granting your patient total-body atherosclerosis will keep you from being caught by surprise when the smoker with coronary artery disease comes in with recurrent monocular blindness, hypertensive crisis, or an elevated creatinine. Think of your patient's personal normal as the cumulative progressing pathology he carries in his body every time he walks in the door of your clinic. Breathless.

Expect every complication of chronic ethanol guzzling in everyone who drinks. Expect the incredible diversity of opportunistic infections in anyone HIV-positive. Expect mental status changes and seizures today or tomorrow in your lung cancer patient. You aren't being a pessimist or a cynic—you're simply letting some differential diagnoses and the natural history of personal disease-bearing run their courses in your head.

When a problem list starts looking too long, weed it out. Does your patient *really* have twelve different diseases, or are they merely subsets of an all-pervasive pathology? Why not put the aortic aneurysm repair, carotid endarterectomy, the coronary bypass, renal artery stent, and the leg amputation together as a single disease—a single challenge for the two of you.

Given an age of 97 years is there *anything* you've put on your patient's problem list that you consider truly *abnormal*? If so, why? Revisit your demographics every few months, Doctor. Become a philosopher.

Your chronic back-and-shoulder pain patient will have other recurrent aches and pains until proven otherwise.

Your migraine patient will have more than one type of headache spread out over decades and may have some other autonomic baggage like irritable bowel and dizziness too. Look for major themes, trends, and personal idiosyncrasies when you're plotting graphs of your patients' destinies in your head.

Don't think of yourself as a lumper, a splitter, or a reducer—but as an abstractionist. Such a serene mindset conserves your energy and frees up your resources for concentrating on the acute scenarios that make your doctoring a world of excitement.

Keep It Simple

Doctor and patient working with new diagnoses are akin to parent and child discussing sex. Address only what is appropriate today. Doctors talk too much. We confuse our patients with all those beloved words we paid so dearly for:

"The medication I'm prescribing for you works at the level of the ion channels of the cell membrane, keeping the calcium ion from passing through and therefore altering the resting membrane potential. Any questions?"

You may be treating a theoretical physicist who has an IQ 50 points higher than yours at your best. But does she have any idea what a beta-blocker's blocking? Where in the world would she have learned such trivia? Even if she's tried to treat her insomnia by reading a physiology text, how would she have picked up a visceral sense of the quirks of her own receptors? And do you *really* understand all that theory yourself? Of course not.

Don't get elaborate. Your patient can deal with only one major new idea in a visit. And that doesn't include taking it home, sleeping on it, looking it up on the Internet, and talking to friends. If what you've just told your patient invokes anxiety, then even less—perhaps nothing—is going to get absorbed, let alone understood:

"Doctor, when I saw you last week I was so worried about my eye. I'm terrified of going blind. I have to apologize, but I didn't understand what you were saying about muscular dystrophy."

"Multiple sclerosis—also known as demyelinating disease."

"Yes, I'm sorry, multiple sclerosis. Now that my eye is better, that's what's got me so upset. I had a friend with

MS—that *is* what you said isn't it? And I watched her deteriorate. It was horrible."

The woman crying in front of you has a Ph.D. in biochemistry and another in engineering. Why didn't she get it straight? Because her experience, knowledge, and vision lie in a world alien to the ways of the dendroglia, that's why. Besides, it's her body and her feelings about what's going on inside it, not yours, Doc.

For the physician *"You've got hypertension, and by the way you're diabetic too"* is a no-brainer. But think of your patient, having to digest his interpretation of what you just said:

I'm a diabetic—just like my brother who died of a heart attack at age forty.

To you, all of this is dry "routine" material:

"Your blood sugar is 250 so we'll be putting you on a medication to lower it, and I'll tell you about the side effects in a minute, and I want you to start monitoring your glucose at home—the nurse will show you how to do that—and I want you to start on this diet. I want you to lose 70 pounds, and your blood pressure's getting up there, so we'll have to watch that and recheck your cholesterol when I see you back next month. Is that clear?"

This is way too much. Too much information, generating too many emotions and memories. Did you notice that glazed look that descended after about ten words of your spiel? You'd be lucky if she understood two percent of what you just said. And that's a generous two.

Today could simply have been diabetes 101—an introduction to blood sugar and its management, with a bit of reinforcement and hands-on performed by your loyal staff. The glucometer and a gentle easing into the enormous challenge of the diet might be all she can handle. Kidneys, feet, eyes, and glucose-tweaking can come later.

One patient started jerking his leg the day he was told he was diabetic. It took six months for us to realize that he was acting out his fear of the surgeon's saw. His diabetic brother had had both legs amputated. Too much scary stuff delivered too soon.

The disease is the easy part. It's the playing out in the body and mind of your patient that requires your sensitivity and wisdom. Don't open up any more disease than you can work with in seven minutes. After all, your patient has to go home and translate every word you say into her language and the language of her body. That's a lot of cultural anthropology and dream material for even the strongest of souls.

Watch your language. How often does anyone use *hiatus* in daily speech? Let alone funny words like *cecum* or *prolapse*? And we haven't even got around to the heavyweights like *myelodysplastic* and *lipoprotein*. Pictures, x-rays, well-done anatomic models can help. Keep these sculptures and graphics out of sight unless you need them. When you bring them out of the cabinet do so as though for the first time. And, in doing so, touch your patient's body to establish surface landmarks and points of reference for your aids.

Avoid theory and avoid the theory-dependent world of molecular biology. Think how long it took *you* to become conversant in *that* lingo. And even now, how many of those channels and receptors do you have a gut feel for? Share your knowledge, your ignorance, and your patience. If that physicist leaves your clinic baffled, let it be openly mutual.

Neutral Monsters

There is nothing wrong with disease. Does cancer know it's cancer? The plague bacillus is a robust bug, not a character in a horror film. Disease isn't the enemy or any other metaphor. It's fire to the fireman or dented fenders to the body worker. It's our thing, our stock in trade.

Despite historical contamination from words like *malignant* and *invasive,* we aren't practicing on the stage of good and evil. Clear the value-laden language out of your dialog. Put your patient at ease by sharing your knowledge with her, not your attitudes. Show her some pictures, describe alternative scenarios, and let her look at that slide under your microscope. She can get the tear-jerking version from *Reader's Digest.*

Patients can't help mixing pathology with emotion. Who among us has the equanimity to separate disease from diseasehood—those elegant mitotic figures from what's growing in your very own breast?

We physicians, though, have a slight advantage in this territory. We've seen some grotesque and chilling stuff. Our patients haven't a clue of our personal inventory of firsthand faces-of-death experience. Use what sophistication you've gained in the arena of pathos to keep disease separate from suffering. And don't let suffering get confused with altered tissue. Remind yourself and remind your patients. They'll be relieved.

If you feel vulnerable from time to time, go see your pathologist, talk to an oncology buddy, or spend an emergency room Saturday night with a trauma surgeon. Your mind will be clearer for it.

Disease is exciting, fascinating, and a continual source of awe and wonder. Its presence sheds light on the human condition and on the peculiarities of this high primate critter of ours. Fear and loathing dull our perception of those exotic cells. Honor disease. It's been around a lot longer than you.

Suffering

Suffering is narrative at its most gothic, the Edgar Allen Poe or Franz Kafka of outpatient discourse:

"I don't know what I'm going to do. No matter what I try, things just seem to get worse. I'm all bound up inside. Maybe if I tried that new garlic and papaya diet it would help me. I don't think anything inside me is working right. I feel so exhausted, like my get up and go has got up and gone. Every ounce of energy is drained out of me. And I'm getting by on about one hour's sleep. I know it can't be any more because I look at the clock and it says one and then two and three. I know my bones don't have enough calcium in them, and it feels like my food's not getting down there right when I get upset. And I shake inside, not like—God forbid—Parkinson's—God, I hope I don't have that too, but like all my organs are vibrating deep inside. And this terrible ringing in my ears! All day and all night. I think it's one of the reasons I don't sleep. I just can't enjoy myself. I try to go out with friends, and we'll be at a restaurant and I'll have to say, 'I hate to spoil your meal but I really think you're going to have to take me back home.' They've been so understanding. I know they care, but they can't help me."

Wow! What rhetoric, what a sense of mainstream medical pulp melodrama you have, my dear.

Most of us are occasional sufferers, and most of our patients limit their suffering to times when they're sick—when there's a disease up front to work with, or when there's a genuine crisis. It's the steady background rumble of dysphoria, the chant of the career sufferer that tests our listening skills.

Don't take the well-seasoned whine personally. Just because you don't enjoy daytime television doesn't mean it lacks cultural value. Recall the reception of the first performance of Stravinsky's *Rite of Spring*—crowds storming out of the theatre shouting and shaking their fists.

Somatizing narrativity is a special way of presenting the self in the world. Practice critical listening when working with the somatic stylist. You might consider some warm-up exercises by listening to radio evangelists, insurance salesmen, and farm reports. This is your opportunity to practice extracting message and content. Adjust the gain on your speaker's hyperbole. Contemplate the colorful images: *How do I, or you for that matter, know what it feels like to have "a thousand little guys with hammers, each one doing his own thing" inside your head?*

"Then what do you do?"

"I just lie down and feel bad"

"Do you fall asleep?"

"No—I just lie there for 8 or 10 hours. . . ."

"But what do you *do* during that time?"

"I just suffer, that's all. I just lie there and suffer."

It has taken a whole lifetime to develop this kind of rhetoric. You can't expect to fast-forward to the disease part without a lot of practice. Listen to the music as though to the work of an avant-garde composer. Sooner or later your ears will become attuned and you'll begin to pick out the melody, the hidden stream of mental activity. Imagine tissue. Think of those models of the Visible Woman and Visible Man while you're listening. Deconstruct those metaphors! Imagine your patient in front of a surveillance camera with the sound turned off, going about the mundane moves of her day. Imagine those bowels, those semicircular canals, that contracting myocardium. Then, take off your analytic hat for a moment and listen to the voice behind the words:

I'm telling you something, Doctor, maybe in a peculiar way, maybe in a way that doesn't suit you, but it's my song, my soul under there. Me.

Dread

When you glance at your appointment book, spot a certain name, and instantly get a queasy shiver running down your spine, it's time-out for a Dread Zap. Somehow, perhaps over the course of several visits, you got yourself backed into a corner, resigned to having to listen helplessly to an unrelenting hundred-decibel whine cum tirade.

"I have 10 incurable diseases and you don't seem to be able to do anything about any of them. And by the way, all those medications you prescribed cost me 500 dollars and they made me so sick I had to flush them down the toilet."

This is what you imagine you're in for. All this and more—based on two or three previous thumbscrew visits that left you convinced that going to medical school was a bad idea. The worst decision of your life.

Dread thrives when we've lost sight of our initial goal of studying people's health and disease in an atmosphere of benevolent neutrality. Somehow we let things slip by us with this patient, and we started doing things we didn't want to do. We found ourselves saying that symptoms would improve when we knew they wouldn't, ordering tests when we knew the normal results would only stimulate further discord, and prescribing meds when we knew they wouldn't work. We failed to constrain, to negotiate, to explore the underlying conflicts that had got translated into global dysphorias long before we ever met.

Dread is always *our* doing, a byproduct of one or two sloppy visits, a little procrastination here, and a little naive optimism there. Usually the dear doctor fails to see certain features of personality conflict lurking on the dark side of her countertransference. Dread grows and expands rapidly in the patient's absence and lets up ever so briefly when your patient no-shows for an appointment.

Aside from preventive medicine—not letting things get out of hand in the first place, or just breaking off the relationship—is there a remedy? Sure, not easy—but sure:

"Mr. Zomata, I was reviewing your records this morning, your x-rays and labs from your previous visits, and reports from the hospital and from the other doctors you've seen."

These lines need to be intoned slowly and solemnly, showing that you've done a lot of thinking about his case. And they're delivered while you're standing—keep the high ground.

"I know you've been feeling bad for a long time, for at least 15 years. I get the impression that nothing that's been done up to this point has given you much satisfaction. You've expressed a great deal of unhappiness with whatever I've done here, and I get the impression you're not too happy with my treatment or, for that matter, my diagnosis. What do you think is going on? What's *your* picture of what I can realistically do for you? In your heart-of-hearts do you believe I can be of any help to you at all?"

Once in a while your dread turns out to be unfounded, and the visit goes smoothly. You're totally surprised. When this happens, replay the session in your head as soon as the patient leaves. Where did your fantasy come from? Could it still be played out at some future visit? Without knowing it, did you do something healthy to avert disaster?

Sometimes all that's needed is ventilation:

"I've heard your symptoms, and you certainly have a lot of them. You've told me about your bad experiences with a lot of doctors—including me. I've done most of the talking today. Why don't you tell me what's going on with you, what you're thinking about right now. How do you feel about all this—your life, your health, and your doctoring with mc? I'd like to hear what you have to say."

If you're going to start over today, then make it start-over day. It's not new symptom day and it is *not* "how are you doing?" day. Nonetheless, you'll sit close to your patient, as always, and you'll perform a focussed exam while you're talking. Dimming the lights and a few seconds of ophthalmoscopic hocus-pocus might just hammer home the point that *you,* at least, haven't lost sight of the initial goal—giving your patient your doctoring best:

"Mr. Zomata, I'm not going to order any more tests today, and I'm not going to prescribe any medications. We're going to take a break from all that. Let's get together in a month. That'll give you some time to think about whether we can continue to work together."

The principles here are to reify what medicine is all about, to demystify his expectations, inject a little gratification delay, and to reclaim your territory, namely doctor-land. To make it work, you have to be willing and prepared to give up the Zomata if necessary, and to have your name added to his list of lousy doctors. Ask yourself if either of you is going to profit from continuing. If both your health and the health of your patient are deteriorating with each visit, then it's time to say goodbye forever.

Remember that there is never a need for dread. In the end, that queasy feeling hasn't a thing to do with your patient. Good timing, courage, and a little humility can just about always save the day. Dr. Frankenstein lacked all three.

Aristotle

One of our Shakespeare professors would walk into class with the front page of the daily paper in his hands, reading a headline disaster story. *Tornado kills one hundred. Tragedy strikes small town.* "Too bad," he'd say, folding the paper. "Too bad, but not a tragedy." Naturally, the whole town hadn't been saturated with a tragic flaw, hubris, or any of the other Aristotelian elements that plagued Oedipus and, much later, Hamlet.

So just how bad can your patient's plight be? After all, your first patient, the cadaver, was dead. *It's got to be uphill from there*, we might think. Wrong. Comes before you today your dear patient bearing newly diagnosed metastatic melanoma. He's in the prime of life when all is comfort and fulfillment and grand plans and sweet dreams. Death is simple, over and out. Dying, though, requires finesse.

The advantage of dying is that it can replace procrastination with projects that may never get tackled. The will, the intimate loose ends in desk drawers, the resolution of secrets, letters to friends, the stuff we dream of doing and never get around to.

You enter the room reading the paper, looking just a tad grim:

"Poor guy, shot right on the street with a shopping bag full of toys for his kids in his hand. Didn't have a chance to say goodbye or to tell them how much he loved them. I'll bet he had some other things he would have wanted to take care of too."

That melanoma is starting to look like a good deal.

So What?

Pain isn't a pain. Pain lies in the same province as vertigo, palpitations, night sweats, and constipation. It's neither good nor bad, nor is it real or all in your head. You'll never know, Doc, what's going on in the crosstalk between your migraineur's thalamus and her frontal cortex. Never.

If your patient brings you a pain narrative, a statement of *being in pain*, then that's sufficient. Don't waste a nanosecond on the erroneous *"I think he's faking"* or its counterpart, *"I think it's real. I think he's really suffering."* The patient who, five minutes ago, was grimacing and contorting on your exam table moaning, "Oh my God, Doc! I just can't stand it. Can't you please do something?," leaves the clinic joking with his kids and lifting them into the back seat of his minivan, headed for the zoo. So what?

It's *pain plus what else?* that demands our vigilance. Headache with fever, belly pain with absent bowel sounds and guarding, back pain with reflex changes, are all red flags. But then the complaint could just as easily have been dizziness or flatulence—dizzy plus *what*? Farts plus *what*?

Those early physical diagnosis sessions brainwashed us into believing that where there's smoke there's fire. We became Pavlovian preparations, knowing that if our dear patient so much as held his hand in front of his sternum and flexed his fingers 2 millimeters he was going to get serial enzymes, EKGs and a cath. Back pain back then was myeloma, and headache was either a brain tumor if it had been there awhile or a bleed if it was "The worst headache of my life." The concept of "essential" pain or "benign" pain was completely lacking in stature, credibility, and glamour. And it seemed to live over there in the neighborhood of "diagnosis of exclusion" that we were never too keen on exploring.

When the patients screamed, we leapt into action, poking and scanning and trying our hand at whatever procedures we could inflict on them in the name of biomedicine. When we came up empty-handed, just having acted out the ritual of the workup was consolation enough. And we could still read and dream about those fascinomas we didn't find.

It was at about that time that we discovered the phrases "ruled out" and "atypical" and "functional," the euphemisms for "not medicine as we know it." We were busy enough with "real" disease to let the ruled outs and the functionals sail off into the sunset—sooner or later to be washed up on the shores of primary care. And now it's *your* beachhead, Doc.

In the course of re-programming our approach to the mystery of pain we need to become *completely* comfortable with splitting off symptomatic from essential pain. It's a vocabulary thing. Use the word *essential* in a pain sentence every day. We like the word *benign* too. Try it as well on for size and feel:

"Mrs. Desphore, what's been going on with that *benign* back pain you've told me you've had for the past 40 years?"

"Benign, Doctor? What do you mean *benign*?"

"I mean that your pain doesn't reflect a disease that's going to cripple you or shorten your lifespan. It's not like your hypertension. Your high blood pressure damages your body, as we've discussed before. Your pain may be unpleasant but it's *benign*."

We are *so* afraid of missing bad disease, so haunted by even the idea of those chilling words: "Doctor, I want to fill you in on what's happened since my last visit."

"Go ahead."

"You know, you've been telling me for a year now that I have degenerative joint disease, and there's nothing that can be done about it except to take pain killers. Well, I thought I'd get a second opinion, so I went to another doctor. She's an expert and she's just wonderful. But she found cancer and she got right on top of it. Since I saw you I've had surgery, and she's started me on chemotherapy and radiation. She says it's pretty far advanced. I just wanted you to know."

Is it not an irony that she's said nothing about her pain? Not a word.

We can't live under a cloud of the fear of missing something. Sure you'll miss a disease some day, but blurring the symptomatic with the essential when you're dissecting a patient's symptoms will only increase that likelihood. Disease is disease and pain is pain. Every time you examine your patient look at her disease and then her pain, separately and together. Essential pain is not second-rate pain. It's just an entirely different beast. Do your work up, but do it *in parallel* with your management of the pain, rather than before or after. In this way the idea of the essential is up front, there from the beginning. Putting off introducing the idea of essential pain until you've exhausted yourself in the pursuit of the organic is a colossal anticlimax and a great source of anxiety for both of you.

It is a peculiarity of the physician mind that we abandon our rich knowledge of the chronic when confronted with the acute. To us doctors, new is always *virgin* new until proven otherwise, the sins of the past overlooked and forgotten as the patient lies there moaning:

"How long have you been having these headaches?"

"About two days, Doc. They just won't quit."

"Have you ever had them before?"

"No, never."

If we resist the temptation to get right into the act of fixing, we can make our lives a *lot* easier. Let's try it again with the same patient.

You enter the room where Helen has thoughtfully turned off the light and let your patient lie down on the examining table with an emesis basin clutched in her hand. You approach and put your hands on her temples, murmuring *very* slowly:

"Going back over your whole life *(pause),* when did you first start having any kind of headaches *(pause),* even if they were *completely* different from what you've been having here recently?"

"Nothing like this, Doctor."

You are *not* going to be put off the scent: "When was the first memorable headache of your lifetime?"

"When I was ten, I used to vomit with them, and I'd get these squiggly lines in front of my eyes. I missed a lot of school. My mom had the same thing. So does my older sister. She goes to a migraine specialist."

Now you're talking.

The rule of thumb with chronic pain of any kind is: *Don't start with the presenting complaint. Start with the lifelong pain pattern.* This is particularly valuable when you find yourself dealing with the patient who wants to establish a connection between a recent disaster and a recent pain. It's going to be close to impossible to get your patient to budge from "I never had anything like this until my car wreck" if you start with the car wreck. Take a deep breath and start with ancient history and hold your ground. The same strategy applies, incidentally, to getting a patient prepped for a lumbar puncture:

"Tell me about headaches. What kinds of headaches of *any* kind have you had over the past 20 years?"

"Oh, Doctor, I've had these terrible migraines. I have to go to the emergency room and get shots for them about once a month."

"We're going to be doing a lumbar puncture. As you know it's quite common to get a headache afterwards. And with your history, I wouldn't be surprised if you get one of your migraines. We'll take extra precautions with you. You'll do fine."

Aren't you glad you asked *before* you started unwrapping that LP tray?

Forget about that diagnosis of exclusion idea when you're working with chronic pain:

"I'm going to order a CT scan of your abdomen because you've never had one before, and you've been having that belly pain for a long time. The CT is very good for detecting tumors and abnormalities in blood vessels, and a number of other diseases. With your symptoms I expect the scan to be normal. I don't believe that your pain is a reflection of active progressive disease in your abdominal organs. I want the CT for a baseline so that if you *ever* have an abdominal problem in the future we'll have a previous study for comparison. Any questions?"

You've poisoned the well and you've held your benign pain ground.

Physicians are almost as afraid of being thought of as insensitive as we are of missing a diagnosis. But sensitivity doesn't take care of the problem. Pursuing the course of chronic pain takes patience, tenacity, and courage. Once you've taken up the challenge, don't back down and don't turn back:

"Doctor, I just can't stand it. Please do something!"

"You've had this for a long time. You've had a lot done. You've had 15 surgeries, and you've been on chronic daily narcotics for 10 years, and the doses keep going up."

"I know, Doc. I know! Can't you do something?"

"Tell me how you feel."

"I'm hurting. Can't you see I'm *hurting*?"

"I know you're hurting. Or you wouldn't be here. Why don't we talk about how you feel? What's going on in your head right now?"

Being sensitive doesn't mean losing your way. You want clarity and truth and you want to progress with your patient's therapy. Kissing the booboo, which might work great for a knee abrasion, isn't what this patient needs. He's gone through it before—over and over, and it hasn't worked.

There is nothing in the Hippocratic Oath that demands we fix pain. There is, though, the implication that we take a dedicated and humane interest in it—that we give it our best shot. There are times when our dialog alone takes some of the horror out of the experience. We must learn to know when that's enough.

Socrates

Get Socratic. WWSD? What would Socrates do? Most of your work in the clinic demands no deep philosophical pondering—the strep throat, the reflux, poison ivy, the ingrown toenail. Thus, with these quick fixes, we chug through the day, forgetting that we have some special tools at our disposal:

"What's your idea of what it would be like to be free of your irritable bowel," might be just the right line for today's despondence. "How is your life affected by the symptom? How does Dave respond to your illness? At the risk of being wrong, what are your thoughts on what's causing your symptoms, regardless of all these doctors' opinions?"

Such a line of questioning requires precise attention to timing. Develop the skill of reading your patient's minute-to-minute capacity for introspection and self-analysis. Take a few chances:

"Do you think we're getting anywhere with your back pain? Do you truly believe that you'll ever be free of the pain? As unpleasant as it is, do you think it serves a needed function for you?"

Know, at least, that you have these options. Why keep the questions to yourself when your dear patient, perhaps from a differing viewpoint, is asking too? She's asking and keeping it to herself.

One of our flock would throw us a pseudoseizure in the waiting room, or when she was an inpatient for some unrelated condition. Once she performed at the very moment we were filling in a form for her driver's license. The pattern was nerve-wracking enough to mention to some psych pals we ran into a few months later. "Has anyone ever asked her why she does it?" all of them wondered. We never had.

Often we don't ask because we don't want to think of ourselves as failing to exact a cure. And we don't want our patients to tell us so either. Swallow your pride. Once you get into a Socratic mode you have a chance to refine the way the two of you discuss the future of her illness. The responsibility may be threatening at first, but your access to the patient's soul can be worth it:

"You're the only person in this room who knows how your dizziness feels. Using any words, or phrases, or comparisons you want, give me some idea of what that spinning's like."

"I don't know, Doc, dizzy. That's all."

Don't give up. Go on to something else that builds transference like: "This has been some ordeal for you, hasn't it. I can only imagine some of the things you've been through. . . ."

Sure you'll get some resistance: "Why are you asking me all these questions, Doc? Why don't you just run some tests and find out what's wrong?" Don't take it personally. Nobody's asking you to swallow hemlock.

Days of Our Lives

Some patient-wrangling techniques we use many times a day. Others may be brought into play once a week or once a month:

"Why don't you describe a typical day in your life, from the moment you open your eyes to the moment you go to bed and fall asleep."

This is most useful when a question like "How has your alcohol intake changed in the past year" doesn't seem to be getting you anywhere. Bring your chair close, get prepared to interrupt, and start taking the pulse if the narrative drifts:

"What time do you get up"?

"Around six."

"And then what?"

"Well, I have a drink. I keep a bottle next to my bed. I reach over and have a drink, and then I get up and go to the bathroom. Then I turn on the television and make coffee. Maybe I'll have some more vodka and read the paper, if there's anything interesting."

"Do you eat breakfast"?

"Coffee, that's all"

"So between six and let's say noon, how much vodka do you drink?"

"Maybe a pint, maybe closer to a fifth—depends on what I'm doing. Like today I knew I was coming over here so I had about a pint. Any less and I'll have a seizure."

"What about the afternoon?"

"That's when I do most of my drinking."

"So that's why you have trouble keeping afternoon appointments?"

"Yeah. I like to stay in pretty much."
Aren't you glad you asked?

Not-so-great Expectations

"I've been to at least 30 doctors for this back pain, and I've tried nonsteroidals and steroids, injections and electrical stimulators, narcotics and muscle relaxants, antidepressants and anticonvulsants and Botox, not to mention acupuncture and six surgeries. And I go to a chiropractor and a massage therapist. Isn't there something else *we* can try, Doctor?"

Beware the word "we", and beware the word "try." As long as you're at it, why not eliminate these words as well as "hope" from your clinical vocabulary? "We" smacks of coercion and conspiracy—we against them. Don't let the word cut you off from the rest of the world, Doc. You may need its help some day.

"We" can barricade your clinic to options other than "We'll just have to keep trying until we come up with something that makes you better." Don't hold your breath. Surrender early. Your patient's words are no longer a presenting complaint, but a declaration of irresolvable misery. There's no room for conventional symptoms-and-signs diagnosis here. He had decided to perpetuate the mystery of his plight long before he arrived for the appointment. Take time out before you launch into another in a series of certain failures:

"What do you think you have to show for all the time, and suffering you've put into your disorder? Do you think any of your treatment has made you any worse? What do you think is eventually going to happen to you? Do you see yourself sitting in a doctor's office ten years from now talking about the same symptoms?"

In this probing, you've sidestepped any pressure to diagnose and treat. Give you and your patient room to breathe:

"You have major health problems—diabetes, hypertension, elevated lipids. These are the areas I think we can do something about. After listening to all you've been through with your back pain, I don't think I can be of much help to you."

Sometimes breaking even is about all you can shoot for: "We've looked at your weight, and how your insulin requirements have kept going up over the last two years. I think this may be about as much as we can do without making some major changes in what you eat. I know that's been a challenge for you."

You're not resigning and you aren't throwing in the towel. You're standing back and looking at the whole landscape.

We all like a challenge, and we all like the picture of giving every patient our best. Sometimes "the best" means freeing a patient up to go elsewhere, if even for a specific part of her care. Bend over backwards when you're involved with illness and disease you know you can manage. But be humble, be a realist, and let her know what's out of your league. And let her know early in the game.

Compliance

Who in the world does what he's told? It's the naive physician who whines about noncompliance, a term you might as well eliminate from your vocabulary. Right now. Compliance is the stuff of paternalism, a one-sided perspective of how your patient is leading his life. Think of the friends and dear ones you've "told" to mend their ways—to lose weight, quit smoking, start going out in the cold to do something aerobic every day. Unless the conversation shifted to matters non-medical, has any one of them listened to you?

Better yet, test yourself. Despite your "knowledge" of the world of medicine, how much of a change have you made in your own diet? What about that colonoscopy, so kindly offered by a well-meaning peer who said he'd do it for free at a time that was convenient for you? What about that brisk walk in the park, or those every-3000-mile oil changes? And your car doesn't require an enema or any born-again changes in the way it drives through life.

The doctors with seemingly compliant patients are bullies. Their patients are browbeaten into submission—terrified about their Haagen-Dazs and forced to lie through their teeth about taking those pills you prescribed. And who wouldn't after surfing the net to discover that they cause sudden death? The compliance bully knows what's right for her patient and goes about setting up a black-and-white scenario in which his destiny reflects the degree to which her orders are obeyed. Hypertension, diabetes, epilepsy, and congestive heart failure are favorites:

"I notice your blood pressure is 260/130 today. Haven't you been taking your beta-blocker, your thiazide, and your

Lasix?? I've *told* you before how important it is *never* to miss a dose."

"Sure, Doc—I took them this morning"

"And your salt intake. What about that diet I gave you?"

"No salt, Doc! I don't eat any salt at all. And my wife doesn't cook with it."

Don't set your patient up. Don't back him into a corner. Don't make him lie to you. Leave him a graceful way out.

"The last time I saw you, I wrote you a prescription for some Lasix. Have you been able to handle it? How about all that extra urine output we talked about? Have there been some days when you've had to skip a dose because you knew you wouldn't be able to get to a bathroom?"

"Sure, Doc—like this morning. I knew I was coming to see you, and it's an hour and a half drive with no rest stops. I couldn't have made it without stopping."

Sometimes we simply bypass the compliance question and bludgeon our way into our patient's life and body. Rather than dealing with the patient squirming and screaming on the table the kindly surgeon has her knocked out and paralyzed.

You're septic? We're going to put in a central line and pump in antibiotics around the clock. No questions? So why are we angry or surprised when the lines get pulled out mysteriously, or when the loyal nurse lets you know she shoved down that nasogastric tube for the third time. You never asked, you never negotiated, and you never explained.

"What do you think about taking some valproic acid on a daily basis to see if it will cut down how often you have your migraines?"

"I've never liked taking pills, Doc. My mother got hooked on narcotics, and she was just out of it all the time. They put her on antidepressants, and she just slept all day. Her doctors put her on everything in the PDR for migraine, and I don't see it ever helped her one bit."

"Valproic acid isn't a narcotic and it isn't an antidepressant."

"I know, I read about it. It's used for epilepsy too, isn't it? I know it can affect your liver."

"What would you like to do with your migraine? Do you think you'd be following in your mother's footsteps if you took medication for your headaches?"

"I just don't want to take any pills. And I've thought about it a lot."

"What if we start looking at your sleep pattern and your diet and maybe how you deal with stress? Do you think that would be worthwhile?"

"Yes. I think stress has a lot to do with it. What about my diet?"

Changing routines is difficult enough. Changing ways of looking at body, health, and life is a long, slow dialog—often painfully slow. Changing your patient's beliefs might never happen. Your patients absorb, ponder, change course, at their own rates. Rarely can you speed up enlightenment.

"Do you think quitting smoking would help you?"

"No, I don't."

"Do you think any of your health problems, like your claudication, COPD, three heart attacks, two strokes, one blind eye are in any way related to smoking?"

"No, I don't. I think you either get diseases or you don't. Smoking has nothing to do with it. I've had three friends who quit, and they got emphysema and heart disease and died within a couple of years. Mom died of breast cancer and she never smoked. And dad lived to be 90 and smoked three packs a day. And he drank too, a fifth of whisky a day for 50 years."

Patients need time to try out ideas and think about big questions: *Do I have any control over my health? Will the changes you've proposed really make any difference in the long run?* Expect resistance. Resistance reveals your patient's style, and it lets you know how your attempts at doctoring are being interpreted. Psychiatrists look at resistance as the raw material of their daily work. Why shouldn't we?

"Everybody in my family is big. They're all diabetic and they all have blood pressure problems. And most of them die of strokes."

"Do you think you have any chance of beating the family tradition?"

"I don't know. Dad never went to a doctor in his life."

"Can you imagine your dad taking medications for his blood pressure? Do you think he would have listened to anyone about his weight?"

"It's hard to say. He was awfully stubborn."

Perhaps you've created some homework, a soul-searching assignment. If nothing else, you have a point of departure for the next visit:

My doctor is looking at a far bigger picture than simply my diabetes. She's a wise woman. I have some respect for what she's trying to do.

So let's get to work.

Backing off on the compliance struggle gets the job done. If it's not your patient's "fault" that his blood sugars are in the four hundreds then it's far easier to enlist his help in upping and downing his insulin. You're not throwing up your arms, shaking your finger, and rolling your eyes. And he isn't cringing in the corner telling you:

"I just can't figure out why my sugars keep going up. I'm doing everything just like you told me, Doc."

Bite your tongue. Go easy. Play dumb if you have to. At this point you need his help more than he needs yours.

"I'm not going to lecture, and I'm not going to scold. It's not my style. And I'm not going to start using words like 'should' and 'have to.' You've come a long way, and I think you have a much better sense of your diabetes than when we first started looking at it. Bring in your glucometer readings and we'll look at them—high or low. Call me if they're out of the range we've been talking about. And let's keep looking at what you *are* eating. You've said you eat a lot of junk food. Why don't we find out what's in that cheeseburger and shake you mentioned. Do a little research. I'm curious. Let me know when I see you next month."

There is a recurrent compliance theme in a lot of religions—*this is how you ought to behave, and these are the cosmic consequences of not doing so.* The simple messages—or commandments, in some cases—get repeated over and over. Yet still there is universal and perennial noncompliance on the part of the folks who truly, madly, deeply believe in the message. And that's from God, dear and glorious physician. Can you do better?

The Wolf

Know the wolf. The wolf looks like a patient, behaves like a patient, and certainly talks a good patient line, but he's a wolf. There's a car out in your parking lot with the engine running and three passengers in sunglasses. The driver is in your office clutching the side of his head and wincing with his mouth in a capital letter *O* telling you how much he hates taking those narcotics: "But Doc, they're the only thing that works."

The woman with the cervical collar, sent by her lawyer, clutches a thick manila envelope: "I just wish there was something you could do for my neck, Doctor. I'm in *so much pain* I had to quit my job."

A she-wolf is she.

The man clutching the loose-leaf binder with color-coded tabs and graphs all pertaining to the dizziness he's used to baffle 75 physicians over the past twenty years wants you to "explain." *Nobody seems to be able to tell me what I really have.* An inquisitive scholar of a wolf is he.

Patients want our services and expect give-and-take and a bit of negotiation from time to time. The wolf brings a prescribed agenda and wants access to what our meritocracy can provide. Patients come to us for fixing, explaining, managing. Wolves want angles. The wolf knows exactly what he wants before he comes to see you, and he has little interest in cluing you in on his deeper needs. Your assessment of his condition is irrelevant: *This is what I want, and I'm going to get you to give it to me.* Once in a while a wolf needs a doctor. Veterinarians know this, and so should we. Treat and return the wolf to the wild. You have given him your doctoring best with clearly defined limits.

Keep in mind that the wolf can be amazingly oblivious to bona fide pathology. Treat treatable disease, document with a passion, and then let him go. The wolf won't get "just a few" Percocets to get him out of the clinic, nor will you be ordering "just one more" futile test. There shall be no reason to return.

Goldilocks was one of the forerunners in wolf management. She used the technique of gonzo confrontation:

"Correct me if I'm wrong, but it looks like you're seeking narcotics. The DEA has really improved their database."

Presented in this way some wolves are polite and will thank you for your time and leave. There are, though, the older wiser members of the pack:

"So let me get this clear, Doctor. You get your kicks from seeing people suffer? You're not going to write for my morphine until I go back to another one of those pain clinics?"

"I'm not going to write a prescription for morphine."

Ever, period. There is no blackmailing an honest doctor. And an honest doctor doesn't do what she doesn't want to do.

For the wolves with paralegal training you'll need something like this:

"You're wanting me to write up a report so you can get money for having been in a motor vehicle accident? How would I go about that? I don't quite understand. . . ." *This doctor is unbelievably clueless.* Ignorance is bliss. She won't be back.

"I had a chance to look over some of the records from your other doctors. You have certainly been thoroughly investigated. I couldn't hope to shed any more light on what's going on with you. I just don't have the expertise."

Be humble and he'll leave. If you take on the lupine baffler as a challenge, hoping to succeed where others have failed, you're in trouble.

We use all sorts of pejorative terms for the wolf: The drug seeker, the crock, the professional patient, the health care overutilizer, and the malingerer. Leave the bad transference and terminology out of the confrontation. Keep it simple. The wolf is not a patient but rather one disguised as a patient. Don't treat him "as though" he were.

Somatomancers

Our first clinical disenchantment, realizing that we can't make our patients fit molecular models, is bad enough. Then come the hoards of patients we can't find in *Harrison's*. Even in the fine print. We know that the wolf will go back to the forest when she discovers that you aren't a veterinarian, a drug-dealer, or a scam artist. But what about the "difficult" patient, the one with the limitless needs and eternally unsolvable sufferings?

Standing before you now is a man who has spent his career in doctors' offices. His symptoms are presented as mysterious, all pervasive, and unsolvable. And that's before you have a chance to say "Good morning, Mr. Dresden." There is extreme and there is radical. This case will require the latter.

You will remain standing throughout the entire encounter, having removed all the chairs from the room ahead of time. There will be no convenient place for him to spread out his notebooks, files, and hand-carried x-ray films. In fact, before he enters the exam room, it might not be a bad idea to strip him of *all* these props and exhibits, whatever he might employ to lay claim to your territory.

It is essential that you spot his master list of impossible questions on entering the room. Sometimes the list is a little piece of paper with tiny handwriting clutched in the hand, and sometimes it's a notebook with a rubber band around it. Grab it. Grab it firmly and with an air of reverence for all the wisdom it contains:

"You have a list of questions? Let's *(now grab!)* take a look" You turn toward your patient, shoulder to shoulder, as though singing together from a hymnbook, and start reading quickly through the list. As you read you touch. "Everything I eat turns to gas." You are quoting, and as you quote you press the belly gently with your other fingertips.

Unfortunately, this reminds him of something:

"For the past ten years when I get excited I feel that there's something stuck in here that's swelling up. You know, like how bread dough rises. . . ."

Put your hand and maybe your stethoscope on his throat and ask for a swallow. Don't permit a nanosecond's lull in your commentary.

Have a notepad in your white coat pocket, pull it out, and make some notes of your own—with just a hint of a furrowed brow. Remember, you're both still standing. Write a prescription if you like and order a test or two if you must. We're in the home stretch. Gather the belongings from your desk or examining table, making contact with his shoulder, and with a circular motion swoop him toward the door:

"Come out with me and we'll make an appointment for next month."

"But I didn't tell you all the details about my gas. What about my gas, Doctor?"

"I'm glad you told me about it. I think I've got the idea."

Now, you perform one last gentle and firm palm-on-the-belly rite: "Things are OK in there. I'll see you next month."

How often are you going to need to do the stand-up radical visit? Maybe two or three times a year. Remember that the function of this unusual exercise, aside from bringing the visit in under your seven minutes, is to give your patient something to think about: *What's the use of going to see my doctor?*

Even on the best of visits, with your most organic patients, that little piece of paper may come up. It's such a universal part of the doctor-patient charade that the nineteenth century French had a word for it: *la malade du petit papier*. Grab it.

Martians

We all read the tabloids standing in the supermarket checkout line. They're not just a guilty pleasure. We have to keep up. Cancer, universal pain, bad sex—all our favorite medical things—are up there in the headlines every week. And cured too. Where else are we going to find out about the latest on arthritis, how to lose two hundred pounds in a week, and the secrets of eternal youth? Certainly drug reps will oblige our pursuit of magic—and throw in samples and snazzy brochures for good measure. But they hound us, and the tabloids don't.

When our patients come to us plastered with magnets, clutching their herbals and downloads from the snake oil website of the month they're telling us: *You're my doctor. I'm suffering, and I can't figure out why, but I keep searching. I want your help.* All this and some personal somatic entertainment. After all, clipping the latest article on aloe enemas can, we imagine, be about as much fun as tearing out a recipe for pound cake. A fine hobby for the viscerally inclined.

Propaganda is propaganda. Television and print ads from the pharmaceutical giants flood us all. We doctors are perhaps the most gullible, caving in to the drug dinners and journal articles touting the latest *prescription* snake oil. We're desperate. Our lists of incurable diseases are considerably longer than those little laundry lists our patients bring us. And our egos, when it comes to not being able to exact a cure, are far more vulnerable. Is it any surprise, then, that we start to believe that those astronomically expensive pills we prescribe actually *do* something? When's the last time one of your patients looked you straight in the eye and told you: "Doc, I can't believe how wonderful the effects of that alpha-blocker are! I just don't know how to thank you. I've completely forgotten that I have a prostate!"

What is it, then, that separates what we do from the world of the tabloids? Medicine, as we know in our hearts, has always been far more trial and error than bench-scientifically sound. And our track record for complicity in foisting placebos on the populace is mind-boggling. So, what right do we have to dismiss bee stings for multiple sclerosis and chelation therapy for sick building syndrome?

The answer, we suppose, is that we're in for the long haul. We hover up there over our patients through thick and thin, weathering fads, glitches, and quirks of fate. We are disease watchers and trenders. Maybe we're guilty of selling prescription snake oil in our weak moments, and quick to believe in what we read in our own tabloids, but we'd like to think our hearts are pure—and at least our mindful hands are warm. Who are you to say what selenium does? Don't be a snob.

Tests Won't Save You

Sometimes your standard patient-wrangling techniques fail, and panic looms. No matter how glued to the chair your patient may seem, don't attempt to pry him loose by ordering tests:

"I don't think there's anything to be concerned about, but *just to make sure* I'm ordering a complete series of x-rays of your bowel and analysis of your stools for parasites."

These words are bound to come back to haunt you. We remember, as if it were yesterday, a note in broad cursive with big loops on pink paper pinned to the door of a well-meaning but naive medical resident:

"Dan, I pooped in the little cup, and I had the upper GI series, the barium enema (whoopie!) and all those blood tests. Now what?"

"Now what?" is right. This is a case of pay me now or pay me later, putting off the dreaded, "You're trying to tell me it's all in my head," to another day when you'll be no closer to an understanding. Nor will you likely, then, be any more in the mood to confront her illness. Instead, you can head off disaster at the pass:

"We've reviewed your detailed history and the results of the physical examination. There are no helpful lab tests or x-rays for the pattern of symptoms you've been experiencing. Let's see how you respond to these medications, and I'll examine you again in two months. We'll adjust your treatment according to how you're doing at that time."

By rendering a disposition today, you won't get that horrible epigastric cramp and the tingle down your spine the next time you see his name on your appointment list.

There is only one reason for ordering tests—the sincere pursuit of getting a clearer clinical picture. Order tests for you and for the disease, not for the patient. Otherwise, you'll forever be backing yourself into the corner of the inevitable: "Doctor, if my CT and my MRI and my EEG and my spinal tap are so normal, then what *is* causing my headaches?" Make it clear that it's you, dear doctor, doing the diagnosing, and that the lab is simply a tool—no more and no less.

Ordering a laboratory test or an imaging procedure requires the physician to create an illusion of exact reasoning, putting the patient and her tests into a perspective that makes sense to her. One of our patients carried a crumpled lab slip stamped with a slightly elevated phosphate level in his wallet for years. He would unfold it every time he saw a new doctor and ask, as though for the first time, what the value meant. None of us knew, which disturbed him greatly.

Visions of the *abnormal* can be mysterious and terrifying. Avoid the word if possible. Carcinoma is far more carcinoma than it is abnormal. Strangely too, a normal test, with some exceptions like pap smears and T-cell counts, is rarely satisfying. There isn't a normal lab in the world that will *ever* comfort a hypochondriac.

The Joy of Discontinuation

It is amazing how much better you can make your patient by getting rid of all the medications you've prescribed for her. Swallow your pride if it was you, and bite your tongue if it was that other doctor who came within a hair's breadth of finishing her off. We can be thankful that the human body functions almost all the time without any drugs at all, and that your patients have a miraculous resistance to being poisoned with prescription meds.

As if by magic, the eighty-seven year old who passed out yesterday (alpha-blocker), got a huge bruise (warfarin) on his forehead (thank God, not a subdural hematoma), and became acutely psychotic (propoxyphene, benzos, and codeine) is sitting up in bed looking the best he has since you first met him—except for the bruise and a full colon. He's had no medications since yesterday morning.

A very proper lady came back with her arm in plaster after starting three new anti-Parkinson drugs the day before. Within two hours of swallowing the pills she vomited, started hallucinating, got terribly dizzy, fell down, and fractured her humerus: "If it's all the same to you, doctor, I'll just leave my little tremor as it is."

How often does anyone die suddenly from a pill-rolling tremor?

Consultations for acute dementia, change in mental status, obtundation, and dizziness are so frequently drug-related that we're in the habit of asking for a cleaning out of the medicine cabinet before we see the patient. Weed that pharmaceutical garden.

These days pills are the answers to everything. They are essential to health, sex, happiness, and immortality. And the more they cost the better they work. Be courageous — just don't prescribe. Remind yourself that your dear patient is going to be triply angry when you stop a drug that made her sick, didn't work, and cost her half a month's house payment.

Preaching

Our patients know before setting foot in the door of your clinic that they harbor great sins of the flesh. Who needs you to say he's 200 pounds overweight? Do psychiatrists make it a point of telling their patients to straighten up and fly right? Yet primary caremongers seem to spend our nights writing sermons on cigarettes, drugs and booze, junk food, and unsafe sex. Not to mention seat belts and sloth.

It is *so* difficult to change behavior. And it's terribly slow. We change at our own rates with the style we've used all our lives. Think, you near-perfect physician, how long it's taking you to shape up. And you still have a long way to go. Dodging hypocrisy can sap your energy.

To tone down your pomposity and to give yourself some headroom, avoid the "I want you to," the "musts," the "shoulds," and the "oughts." Stand in front of your bathroom mirror and shout out "My God, is that sick! You should be ashamed of yourself! You've just got to stop doing that!" until you're laughing so hard you can't go on.

Facts speak for themselves. Talk about your patient's perception of her body and her risks for developing disease, and throw in a few numbers:

"If we can get your blood pressure into the 130/80 range your chances of having a heart attack or a stroke go down by close to 50%. We've talked about your mother's stroke twice this year. I think it's realistic to get your blood pressure down in that range. What do you think? What do you think is the hardest part about all these changes?"

Don't judge, don't compare, and stay away from the world of the *abnormal*. Instead, get a detailed picture, perhaps over the course of three or four visits, of the facts of your patient's day-to-day life. Find out how those six thousand calories get in there, how a half-gallon of vodka gets rationed out over the course of a day, between naps and coma. Little by little both shame and the edited version of the "occasional drink" and the "just social drink" disappear. Treat behavior in a matter-of-fact manner. At the moment you're walking around inside your patient, comparing him to no one.

Get ready for the truth and accept it with grace and restraint. It can be shocking when your well-compensated CEO cocaine addict starts telling you about seizures, chest pain, and the acute psychoses he's been through with a $500 a day habit. Keep your cool, don't shake your head, roll your eyes, or mutter "unbelievable." What you wanted was a clear idea of what's going on, and he told you. Now get to work.

Your patients are going to change or not change the patterns of their lives at their own paces and on their own terms. Rarely does it matter what they've read, what their closest friends have told them, or how many times physicians have confronted them. If your patient's daughter hasn't got anywhere with "Mommy, I don't want you to die. Why don't you quit smoking?," what do you think you can do, Doc? You can talk, you can describe what's going on in your professional head, and you can provide a safe and private place for her to do some figuring out of her own. Be patient. Your commitment to her health is power enough. Think Gandhi.

Panic Button

It's an emergency if your patient thinks so. Don't waste a microsecond or a single one of your precious cardiac myofibrils:

"If you've had this pain for 20 years, then why in the world are you calling me about it at midnight?" On a holiday, too, Doc.

It may not be terribly easy for your patient, either. It's kind of humiliating to pick up that phone. Even if your patient went to medical school, you can't expect his sense of urgency to reflect astute, cold-blooded diagnostic acumen at the end of a long day of lifting cinder blocks. Take a deep breath, be patient and attentive, and portray no weakness. Bite your tongue.

There are, of course, things you can say. " Mr. Whinhardt, what changed today? I'd like to get a clearer picture of what's happened to your pain in the past 24 hours. I know you've had eleven back surgeries and been in the hospital a lot of times with this pain. What's different about it today?"

Make it clear that you have the talent to put his present situation in a larger context. Let him know that you remember his whole history, and do so when you have your hands on his sacrum. Be circumspect and let him know it. The emergency, in the end, is what's rolling in the door at the moment. Enhance your cool by letting your patient do the whining. All of it.

Your Study

Study the forty or so acute curable diseases that can kill your patient, the ones you never want to miss. Pneumococcal meningitis, ectopic pregnancy, subdiaphragmatic abscess, herpes simplex encephalitis, and ischemic bowel will get you started. If a new one occurs to you in the middle of the night, add it to the list. These are the diseases to know backwards and forwards in all their presentations, particularly the unusual and atypical forms. Know their habits, their demographics, and their varying modes of onset. Program your indices of suspicion for these beasts according to your population. Read all the case reports of the top forty you can get your hands on. When the weather's bad, go to the subspecialty literature for touch-ups every couple of months. Study comorbidity, disease associated with disease, so that if you're lucky enough to stumble on one diagnosis you won't miss the ones that are going along for the ride.

Read therapeutics when you're tired, and read it out of sight and sound of the drug reps, perhaps in the bathroom. Look for the fine print at the bottom of clinical trials, letting you know that the product is brought to you by a generous donation from the people who are about to tell you how well it works. Equate drug brochures with tabloids. Read the alternative therapy literature. Your patients certainly do.

Study the dermatological manifestations of systemic disease. The pathology is right there, staring you in the face. You already know how embarrassing it is when your patient pulls up his shirt and points at a blotch or a bleb:

"Doctor, I'd like to show you something. Would you mind telling me what this is? I've had it for about ten days, and I've been putting cortisone cream on it, and it just keeps getting worse."

Study psychiatry, particularly depression, variations on the anxiety theme, somatoform disorders, and the DSM categories of our commonest problem patients. The personality disorders, particularly the borderline and passive-dependent are high on the list.

When you want a bigger picture, study pathology. It's like going for a hike or taking a cold shower. It instills humility and will never let you down. If you want to study God, then study sacred texts. If you want to get at the heart of medicine and take a break from the media-driven world of populist and industry-driven disease mongering, then read what the diseased body looks like under the microscope. The perspective is always refreshing.

Atypical Horses

Looking for rare diseases in our clinic isn't a totally bad idea. All we have to do is set the zebra trap out in the waiting room and let the unsuspecting creature wander in. *This may look like a zit, but on the other hand it could be a lethal midline granuloma* is the right spirit. The zebra hunter, with his high-powered scope, soon develops an eye for seeing the panic attack as a case of acute cerebral lupus. Plain old migraine is surely temporal arteritis, and yesterday's bad potato salad is an attack of acute porphyria.

The sincere zebra hunter is akin to the amateur entomologist who, with great patience and dedication, has managed to capture 6,000 species of bugs in a hundred square feet of suburban back yard. Vigilance, a keen eye, and the drive to expand the collection work together. And it helps to read the bug journals.

Zebras are not atypical horses. More important, perhaps, than capturing the exotic is recognizing the variants on the common: endocarditis as weakness, pulmonary embolism as dizziness, and ectopic pregnancy or ischemic bowel as sudden collapse. Uncommon presentations of common diseases occur commonly. Read those exhaustive reviews of the common diseases. That's where the atypical horses reside. There and in your waiting room. Do the math.

If you choose to hunt zebras, do so as a hobby — and have a sense of humor about it. We all know the physician who runs her clinic as though she's on a safari:

"Although it may look like prickly heat, I wouldn't jump to the conclusion that it isn't mycosis fungoides. We'd better let the patient know what we're suspecting."

Not just yet. Keep your zebra-hunting a private matter. Do it after hours. Reading esoteric medicine makes you a better if stranger doctor. Let only your very closest friends know of your kinky hobby and your most recent stalkings. And don't tell the horse you think he's a zebra. At least not until you get the biopsy back.

What Do You Want?

You want to wake up every morning for the next 30 years looking forward to going to work at your day job of doctoring. You want to have fun seeing those patients, and you want to turn off the doctoring circuits at the end of the day and go home to a peaceful, joyful other life. Keep the goal in mind: *I want a serene and fulfilled life.*

Some physicians believe it's their duty to suffer under the enormous burden and responsibility of their patients' fates in the universe of disease. We know them, the docs who talk about their exhaustion, carry two or three pagers and a couple of cell phones, and don't get home until midnight. They've mastered the look of looking like war heroes staggering in off the battlefield. They think misery is cool. To the untrained eye it *does* look good. In the movies.

This physician subspecies forever reminds us that doctoring is a form of divine intervention and far more important than having a life. "My patients need me" is their motto. Learn this from them: If a patient needs you rather than needing health care then you've arranged it that way. You've set yourself up.

One of our psychiatrist colleagues got all offended every time a particular patient had an anxiety crisis and ran off to a social worker for counseling rather than calling him in the middle of the night. He should have been thankful — to both his patient and the social worker. Be humble. Give up being special. Give your peace some room to expand.

Don't wait until you're exhausted and discouraged to ask for a consultation. There are fellow physicians who are far better than you, Doc. Why? Because that one case in a lifetime of dermatomyositis you're struggling with is someone-out-there's daily bread and butter. And that someone's got a whole flock of connective tissue oddities in her practice, maybe a whole barn full. That's what she does, Dr. Dermytes, day in and day out. But are you going to send her an aortic stenosis? As if.

So is it with you, dear and glorious physician. Medicine is what you do. Those once in a decade moments of perceived glory can be seductive. Don't take yourself seriously. Take the work seriously. Be humble, keep moving, and the peace will come.

Everybody dies, you and all your patients. All relationships end. Would you want it any other way? If you think you're dealing with chronic now, how about for eternity? Just imagine what those rheumatoid nodules and stasis ulcers would look like in *another* 60 years. And how about that plaque-encrusted aorta? Don't take it personally.

Get a copy of Miles Davis's *Kind of Blue* and listen to *So What?* whenever your grandiosity comes creeping around the corner. Go to your art museum and do the classical sculpture room—or Andy Warhol. Think *Dead Poets* if you must. Read Samurai philosophy to build up your strength—the *Book of Five Rings* and the *Hagakure*. Your life's work may, in the end, be insignificant, but right now, while you're caught up in the furious action of doing medicine, you need all the heavy hitters you can recruit.

You want the image of every one of your patients to get enhanced with each visit. And you want what you do with them to get easier each time rather than more oppressive. Keep expectations earthbound. Promise nothing but being there. Not being there "for you," just being there. You want to hover rather than grapple:

"Let's take a look at it. I'd like to get a clearer idea of what's going on with you. I'd like to see how you respond to A and B."

Here you've given yourself some emotional and intellectual distance without being a cold fish. Compare the approach to "I hope I can help you. . . . This should make it better. . . . I guess we'll have to try something else."

Portray no weakness. Stay neutral and stay cool. You are *not* Dr. Mom.

You want to conserve energy for play. Keep it simple. As an experiment, make a few recordings of your own conversations. If you're brave enough, videotape. Edit mercilessly. Look at what a windbag you are! And, on a bad day, pretty close to insufferable. Confront yourself as if you're a vicious film critic doing her thing. Cut the crap. You'll love it.

Make each visit into a one-act play with a beginning, middle, and end. You want your clinic to flow as smoothly as the course of a great drama, or, for that matter, a great river. Work with achievable goals rather than hopes, and let the patient know which is which. Finish today's business today. Never put off delivering bad news or dealing with dissatisfaction to the next visit. It can only get worse.

You want to minimize liability. Keep your notes detailed and free of weak ambiguities and meaningless fluff like "doing better . . . no new complaints . . . within normal limits." If your goals start looking fuzzy, or you think you have a nefarious motive on your hands, make your notes longer and more comprehensive and include as many direct quotes as you can. Make the length of your notes inversely proportional to the amount of hard-core organic disease on the table. It's often the psychosomatic stuff that muddies the water. That's when you write a progress note that reads like *War and Peace*. The ruptured viscus takes about eight words.

Continually reassess your rapport: *"What's your opinion of how you're doing"* may give you a chance to look at an unhappy camper's opinion of your treatment before things get out of hand. Portray commitment. If you detect friction, make time for a summit conference with your patient *immediately*—a few minutes to clear the air and look at your relationship.

You never want to be unhappily surprised. Don't get in a rut with diagnosis or treatment. For every "common things happen commonly" spend a five seconds imagining "the next one will be the first one." Get in the habit of changing perspective while you're in the midst of the exam. *I have seen her 15 times and I have never seen her before.* You may run into a day of 30 patients with the flu, and out there in the waiting room sits another chills and fever with a cough. Pneumococcal pneumonia, she is. Or would you prefer tuberculosis, Doctor?

You want to be whatever it means to be a good physician. That's easy. Make every visit a case study. Think *Case Records* in the *New England Journal of Medicine*. Don't lapse into informality. If you've been caught up in the mental drone of managing your patient's symptoms for the past five minutes, flip that switch in your head, and do sixty-seconds of her as a case study before you turn her loose. We blow diagnoses when we're distracted, biased, and feeling rushed, far more often than when we're ignorant of the disease.

Every patient has a story you haven't heard. Every patient has a clinical finding hiding inside that you haven't uncovered. Listen. Look. And it doesn't matter to what or at what. A strange fingernail? Tonight you dust off the fingernail book. Your patient doesn't have to know. Think to yourself: *If I were to do an autopsy on my patient today, what would I find?* Keep you on your toes.

Grunge

We don't know how the Haggard Look got started. The successful doctor is supposed to keep "impossible hours," be plagued with interruptions, and never have any "time to herself." She has to be on the go, and on the run—constantly in the midst of something more important than living her life. And we all have to know it.

Surgical residencies brag about their divorce rates. Doctors can't get through the day or night without constantly being paged or called, all decked out with two or three beepers and phones. Wearing scrubs in public and the actors studio look of care-worn exhaustion remain in fashion year after year.

Stereotypes are amusing if they work to our advantage. The disheveled look of beatific detachment in philosophy professors probably gets them tenure. Climbing ladders covered in soot is great advertising for the chimneysweep. Boots on the fishmonger assure us the salmon's fresh. But *doctors*? What in the world do *we* have to prove? Why in the world should we go out of our ways to act miserable? Why should we con our families into going around muttering "He's never home—he works *so* hard!"? Are we *ashamed* of something?

Maybe it started in school when we would compare whines on how many admissions we had that night, and how many codes we'd run, and what a difference we made in all those patients who were crashing. And we'd wear surgical masks pulled down and make sure we had some blood on our scrubs and neglect combing our hair too well. Let's not forget, too, those attendings who'd ham up the grunge image to the max. Ah! What nonsense!

This thing we do is not coal mining. It isn't logging or tuna fishing or working our knuckles to the bone in a sweatshop. If you look strung out, there's something wrong. If you keep getting home late, you've arranged it that way. If you've taken up whining, then it's time to figure out how to turn it around. Unless you're a masochist.

Certainly there *is* such a thing as a long day, but that's about it. It's not a long day of throwing hay bails or sweeping mine fields or diving for sponges. It's a long day in a skilled trade with a huge support system. There's a difference between being pleasantly tired, and portraying yourself as the walking embodiment of all the cares of the world. Make the distinction daily. Medicine is not *that* big a deal, and certainly not worth grunging about. If pasting up a Derelict Rock album cover next to your medicine cabinet is going to help cure the habit, then by all means, paste.

Sleep in. Cook a lovely meal. Work out. Meditate deep into your soul. Get away. Love a partner. Commune with nature. Read philosophy. Put on formal wear and go to a concert. Swim. Do yoga. Restore that house. The human race and all its woes can get along just fine without you. Forever.

The Mountain Top

How much of me do I want to devote to being a physician? How much of the next 30 years of my life am I going to be caught up in the act of doctoring, reading medicine, answering that phone? What fraction of a 24-hour day am I going to devote to the role? How close do I want to be to my patients? What am I going to give them, and what am I going to refuse to give? What buffers do I want to put between us? When will I say goodbye?

Am I going to do the Doctor Thing? Am I going to belong to the Doctor Club and have a Doctor Spouse and Doctor Kids and drive a Doctor Car? Am I an Aristocrat, a Petit Bourgeois Soccer Mom, or an Intelligensiac? A Nomadic Shaman? If I do hang with the Doctor Subculture, do I have an escape route? Am I luring those I love into a Paramedical Lifestyle? How private and mysterious a life do I want?

Is Medicine my religion? Do I hold what I do sacred? Have I answered to a higher calling or is this simply my skilled-trade day job? Have I suffered and sacrificed so that I can be or must be a Martyr or perhaps a candidate for Sainthood? And shall I continue to suffer in order to flesh out my persona? How do I deal with the realm of disenchantment?

Where does my passion lie? How much of my soul is The Doctor? Could I walk out of doctoring gracefully, peacefully, on a moment's notice, and never look back—only to embrace a whole new enchanted life of designing furniture, developing a vineyard, photographing butterflies?

How much baggage shall I carry? Can I travel light? How tied up in a network of referrals and hospital privi-

leges and buildings and equipment and staff do I want to be? Where do I want to live? Forever? Do I want to surround myself with objects? How many? How easily can I throw things away? Does debt bother me?

How much stamina have I? And how shall I conserve it? What about attention span, exhaustion, the specter of futility? How shall I live with stress? What about my body? What gives me pleasure? How long do I want to do what I'm doing? And if I'm maimed?

At some point in a year of seeing patients you'll be ready for the mountaintop. Pack your questions, comfortable clothing, notebook, and music. It will take two days—one to do your thinking, a night to sleep on it all, and the next day to put your ideas together. These will be the most important and likely the most difficult two days of your life in medicine.

Think of the poets, philosophers, and leaders who've gone before you. You'll be alone and you won't be alone. Leave only the world and your contact with it behind. Plan good food. Stay sober. Take aerobic breaks from your pondering. Meditate. Push your mind to its limits—you're good at that. Think well and dream well.

Could it be the shore, the forest, the abandoned warehouse in Rome? Could it be the cliffs, a riverbank, a cave among abandoned ruins? Of course—it's going to be your life for the rest of your life, Doc. So make it beautiful.